DOCTORS' ORDERS

What 101 Doctors Do to Stay Healthy

DOCTORS' ORDERS

What 101 Doctors Do to Stay Healthy

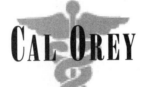

CAL OREY

Foreword by
Julian Whitaker, M.D.

TWIN STREAMS
Kensington Publishing Corp.
http://www.kensingtonbooks.com

TWIN STREAM BOOKS are published by

Kensington Publishing Corp.
850 Third Avenue
New York, NY 10022

All Kensington titles, imprints and distributed lines are available at special quantity discounts for bulk purchases for sales promotions, premiums, fund-raising, educational or institutional use.

Special book excerpts or customized printings can also be created to fit specific needs. For details, write or phone the office of the Kensington Special Sales Manager: Kensington Publishing Corp., 850 Third Avenue, New York, NY 10022. Attn. Special Sales Department. Phone: 1-800-221-2647.

Twin Streams and the TS logo Reg. U.S. Pat. & TM Off.

ISBN 0-7582-0130-3

Designed by Leonard Telesca

First Trade Printing: September 2002
10 9 8 7 6 5 4 3 2 1

Printed in the United States of America

I dedicate this book to my two dearest friends—Dylan, my fun-loving Brittany, and Kerouac, my literary cat—who taught me the art of achieving health and wellness (as did the 101 doctors) by constantly feeding the mind, body, and spirit.

Contents

Acknowledgments

I'm a fan of doctors seen on the big and the little screen. The dedicated physicians on the television series *ER* and the compassionate doctor in the unforgettable film *Patch Adams* (based on a true story) fascinate me. But I'm an even bigger fan of the 101 real-life doctors whose advice appears in these pages, and I'm grateful to them for passionately sharing their knowledge of health.

I thank all the doctors who encouraged me to write this book. And I will remember the understanding ones who have written their own books and who nudged me to stick with it despite the temptation to ditch the "monster project." I know now that it was worth going the extra mile.

Foreword

The idea to go on the quest to discover exactly what 101 doctors do to stay healthy is as good as it gets. And as a physician who helps people achieve health and wellness, I know firsthand that there's a revolution going on in medicine today that will affect the way you take care of yourself tomorrow.

As a longtime doctor of alternative medicine, as well as the new integrative medicine, which is the combination of alternative treatments and standard medical treatment, I am often asked why I took the "road less traveled" in medicine.

I certainly didn't set out to be unconventional. Good formal medical education, which I received and for which I'm grateful, is important, but there was something to come that was far more important to my career as a doctor.

It took place one evening when I was working in the emergency room during my residency at the University of California at San Francisco Medical Center. A young woman came in with a sprained ankle. As I tended to her injury, I was amazed by how healthy she was—so healthy, in fact, that her eyes actually sparkled. Doctors rarely study optimal health, and usually don't advise their patients how to achieve it.

I learned that this woman sold vitamins and took them herself, and as a result of this unforgettable encounter I personally began taking vitamins. More importantly, I began learning all I could about nutritional and natural therapies, subjects often ignored by medical schools. I soon became convinced that these approaches, which drew upon the body's own healing powers, held more potential than prescription drugs and surgery for preventing disease and restoring health.

In 1976, I went to work at the Pritikin Longevity Center in southern California. Then, for the first time in my medical career, I saw patients get well not as a result of dangerous drugs or risky surgical procedures, but through the power of diet and lifestyle changes.

But I believed that there was more that could be done to reverse disease and achieve optimal health. I continued my education, with the goal of discovering safe and effective solutions to common health problems of modern life—heart disease, diabetes, arthritis, and more.

In 1979, I launched the Whitaker Wellness Institute Medical Clinic to share my knowledge with patients. Since its genesis, over twenty-five thousand patients have benefited from the program's diet, exercise, nutritional and herbal supplementation, and lifestyle changes. And they've proven that doctors—like the ones in this book—who practice optimizing health and preventing illness can help you live longer and healthier lives.

In *Doctors' Orders: What 101 Doctors Do to Stay Healthy*, Cal Orey will reveal to you the secrets of leading doctors, mostly nutrition-oriented like myself, who have reaped the benefits of using alternative medicine or integrative medicine.

Come along on this amazing journey and meet inspirational doctors who share their insights for healing themselves, their families, and their patients with the ultimate healthful touch of preventive medicine to help you achieve twenty-first-century wellness.

—Julian Whitaker, M.D., author of *Reversing
Hypertension, The Pain Relief Breakthrough,
and Dr. Whitaker's Complete Guide to Natural Healing*

Preface

One afternoon I lay in bed, cozy in my cabin in the California Sierras, suffering from writer's block. Brain dead, I turned on a television news program. Suddenly, I was listening to an amazing story about a college student who had interviewed more than 80 cardiologists for his thesis. His ambitious feat inspired me.

I thought, "What if I interviewed doctors—all types—and wrote a book about their health habits?" It would be fascinating to probe medical experts about what they do for their own health. I would boldly ask, "How do you prevent illness and disease in yourself? Do you really do what you advise your patients to do?" I could find out how the docs (specialists could talk about their field of expertise) stay healthy from head to toe. It was a splendid idea!

Imagine talking with doctors, dozens of them, and finding out their personal health information! But how many doctors? My enthusiastic editor, Lee Heiman, suggested interviewing 10. "But that's not enough!" I darted back. Even 50 seemed mediocre. If I doubled the amount I could get second opinions (free of charge!). It was the number 101 that clicked in my head. Yes! My idea "What 101 Doctors Do to Stay Healthy" quickly turned into a thumbs-up project that I was ready to tackle.

The goals for this book were twofold: I wanted to learn how

to take care of my own body better and to let readers in on the goods. Rather than wait for an illness or disease to strike, I could seek the pros' strategies to prevent allergies, colds, cancer, and other maladies. The doctors—my subjects—were to be my role models for achieving a healthier and longer life.

My inspiration grew from the doctors' wealth of medical experience and their dedication to helping people's wellness. Some of the doctors are media stars; others are celebrated by their patients and successful work. But each one became my muse as they shared their secrets to good health and well-being. I discovered, one by one, that these 101 men and women of all ages are real people. They struggle with potential and actual health problems just like everyone else. And they do their best to embrace good health.

As I became their enthusiastic pupil, I unconsciously and consciously incorporated some of their diet, exercise, and lifestyle habits into my own daily routine. More fish, less fat. Less stress, more humor. Regular workouts and regular medical exams. And so I resolved to do more and more as they do for my health's sake and peace of mind.

These 101 doctors have given me the key to being a healthier and happier person—inside and outside. And I have discovered that we all have the power to take control of our body, mind, and spirit. These are timeless health secrets of doctors willing to open up and tell it like it is. These are real doctors, and their words of wisdom are worth a million doctors' visits.

The Healing Power
of Doctors

As I grew up in San Jose, California, during the 1960s, the world of health took shape for me on television. I played hooky from school so I could stay home and watch television. Any program (or book) about medical stuff intrigued me, a wannabe writer with a wild imagination. I watched spellbound as the handsome humanitarian Dr. Kildare, played by Richard Chamberlain, cured patients of all manner of diseases. My middle-class neighborhood was a safe place that led me to think that health and wellness came easily to people in my world. But things changed.

Twenty-five years later, there I was, a health journalist writing in the San Francisco Bay Area, interviewing doctors nationwide about the scourge of disease. What's more, reality hit because illness, by this time, had touched my own family, friends, and a past professor or two. I noticed, however, that some of the diseases might have been prevented by lifestyle changes—but it was too late.

Well, these days doctor reality shows such as *Doctors' Diaries* and *Women Docs* intrigue me. On television, doctors are seen as smart, dedicated, and passionate. And as I interviewed 101 doctors from coast to coast (including Hawaii, Canada, and England), it became clear that doctors really *are* like that. The physicians I interviewed are devoted to helping mankind.

This book reveals the incredible power of real-life doctors who have learned how to balance the body, mind, and spirit. The power of health is not something to take for granted, nor does it always come easily. But living healthier and longer can be achieved. These 101 doctors and their stories prove just that.

THE DOCTOR'S LEXICON

Title	What It Means	What They Do
D.C.	Doctor of chiropractic	Provides treatments based on the premise that the spinal column is linked to the nervous system, which affects the total body.
D.D.S.	Doctor of dental science or dental surgery	Diagnoses and treats diseases of the teeth, gums, and related structures of the mouth, including repairing and replacing defective teeth.
D.M.D.	Doctor of dental medicine	Practices dentistry.
D.O.	Doctor of osteopathy	Considers your body structure (your bones and muscles) and the rest of your body functions to operate together. Does everything an M.D. can, including prescribing drugs, performing surgery, and admitting you to the hospital.
D.V.M.	Doctor of veterinary medicine	Diagnoses and treats diseases in animals.

M.D.	Doctor of medicine	Practices general medicine or a specialty such as psychiatry or opthalmology. Prescribes drugs, performs surgery, and admits you to the hospital.
N.D.	Doctor of naturopathic medicine	Treats health problems by assisting the body's natural ability to heal using such modalities as herbal medicine, acupuncture, and nutrition.
O.D.	Doctor of optometry	Examines eyes and prescribes glasses or contact lenses.
Ph.D.	Doctor of philosophy	Performs psychological research and therapy. (Psychiatrists diagnose and treat emotional and mental problems.)

DR. MINDELL'S SUPPLEMENT APPROACH

EARL MINDELL, PH.D.

Dr. Earl Mindell, one of my health mentors, believes that nutrition-oriented doctors are more apt to practice what they preach than conventional physicians. Why? "Because they're more open-minded. They know that there is more than one way to do things." And the majority of the 101 doctors in this book are special, says Dr. Mindell, because they have taken a different path to staying healthy.

Is Dr. Mindell personally taking better care of himself today than he was 20 or 40 years ago? "Are you kidding me? When I was in my mid-twenties I had my own pharmacy. I was working 15 hours a day, had a terrible diet, and was under incredible stress. What did I know?" he says.

What was a terrible diet to Dr. Mindell? "I was eating high fat, high sodium, high sugar," he told me and pointed out that he made a turnaround during 1965 and 1970. "I was under incredible work stress. We had a pharmacy in California that was open seven days a week from nine in the morning until midnight. And then we took night calls from midnight until nine. My associate seemed to be able to overcome stress better than I could. I asked him, 'What do you do?' and he answered, 'I take vitamins.'

"A lightbulb went on, because my mother would always give my father and me a vitamin supplement. I had gotten out of the habit of taking it when I was going to pharmacy school. I started taking a multiple B complex, mineral, and antioxidant. I felt tremendously better."

Today Dr. Mindell is pro-supplements. "In today's toxic environment anyone who doesn't take a supplement is foolish. It's very difficult to get all of the nutrients from our diet," points out the doctor, who also works out three times a week (treadmill, machines, and free weights) and has a personal trainer.

Here are some of the supplements that Dr. Mindell takes himself.

THE DOC'S SUPPLEMENT LIST

Supplement	What It Does
Multivitamin-and-mineral supplement	This combination of nutrients works to keep the body at its optimal health
DHEA	This natural hormonal substance stalls aging and lowers the risk of developing cancer

Ginkgo biloba	This herbal supplement enhances memory
CoQ_{10}, garlic, hawthorn	This combination of a nutrient and herbs helps strengthen the heart
St. John's wort	This herb helps combat stress

Safety Smarts: Ginkgo biloba: Do not take more than 240 mg, since it may cause dermatitis, diarrhea, and vomiting. Do not use it with blood-thinning medications, aspirin, or nonsteroidal anti-inflammatory medicines (NSAIDs). Garlic: Do not use garlic before or after surgery (it's a blood thinner). If you are already taking blood-thinning medicine or aspirin, consult with your doctor first. Hawthorn: Consult with your doctor before using hawthorn, especially if you have low blood pressure. St. John's wort: It may cause sun sensitivity. Do not mix with other antidepressants.

GETTING PERSONAL

According to Dr. Mindell, if you are not taking any vitamins or minerals, especially if you are a baby boomer woman, like me, you are making "a big mistake." Why? "Because as a woman you should know that there is no way you're going to get enough minerals such as calcium and folic acid in your diet. And 48 to 52 is menopausal time, and if there is any time you need a supplement is *now*."

He adds, "I hope you eat soy foods because that is a good way of overcoming the menopausal symptoms. Find tofu, miso soup, and tempeh. Those are good sources of soy that are really easy to take." As I heard the doctor's words, I recalled that he is the one who motivated me years back to dump diet soda and switch to spring water, which has helped me to be a stronger woman with stronger bones.

I asked, "So if I stay on this anti-supplement kick, like millions of other people, will I not achieve wellness and longevity?" Dr. Mindell answered: "What you're saying is, 'I've got an automobile that I bought that I'm not going to take care of. I'm going to keep driving it. I'll wait till it has problems and then I'll take it in and see what's wrong with it.'" In other words, plenty of people, like me, are healthy but ignore doing maintenance because everything seems okay.

Dr. Mindell adds, "We're being brainwashed to know only about sickness. We are ignorant about wellness. We don't know how to take care of our bodies. We only know what to do when we have a problem. When you have a problem you'll call 911 or go to the emergency room and they will send you back until the next problem."

And Dr. Mindell, a doctor whom I truly respect and have interviewed for years, turned out to be right on the money. I had a frightening health wake-up call a few months later.

One morning I was on stress overload: no balanced breakfast, no supplements, disrupted sleep the night before, and work demands piling up. Around 11:30 A.M. I felt dizzy, my vision was blurred, and my heart raced. I quickly fled outside. Thoughts of heart attack or stroke were haunting me. My younger brother called 911.

When the paramedics arrived they took my blood pressure: 158/100. My pulse was too fast and I was frightened as a jackrabbit. A few tests later, my diagnosis: a panic attack. It was my first and hopefully my last. However, because it hit like a bolt of lightning, I have since then begun to s-l-o-w down and try and do as the 101 doctors do. I am learning how to use preventive health maintenance to balance my body, mind, and spirit.

101 DOCS PRACTICE WHAT THEY PREACH

For centuries, doctors like Dr. Mindell have indeed been practicing what they preach and telling people like me how they personally stay healthy. But with the fascination with modern drugs and medical procedures, many of those preventive strategies are ignored. Now, worldwide, an exciting reawakening is occurring, and many of the 101 doctors I interviewed have also experienced turning points in their lives and have turned to the process of healing naturally.

Dr. Harold G. Koenig, the director of the Duke University Center for the Study of Religion/Spirituality and Health, has seen thousands of patients who have successfully beaten disease by the healing power of faith.

Dr. John McDougall advocates the use of nutrition to reverse the effects of heart disease and obesity. He reports that a healthful low-fat, high-carbohydrate diet could cut the risk of disease in half. And that's not all.

SECOND OPINION: SETTING IT STRAIGHT WITH DR. THOMAS

JACK THOMAS, D.O.

Nowadays in the twenty-first century it is not uncommon for people to seek a second opinion, whether it's about their car or their health. "A second opinion is in order if there is any question (by the physician or patient) about the planned course of treatment," explains Jack Thomas, D.O., who practices family and internal medicine. So, if there is any doubt about your health, a second opinion is indeed something to consider.

"The key is that the patient needs to develop a rapport with their primary care doctor with good trust on both sides—a friendship," explains Dr. Thomas. In fact, he points out that people who trust their doctor are more apt to follow his or her recommendations. However, despite our connection with our primary care physician, sometimes we need to seek another option for treatment.

"If you intuitively have any doubts," says Dr. Thomas, "then that is the time to consider getting a second opinion." That means if what a doctor tells you just doesn't sound right, it may be time to seek another doctor's opinion.

One example: After my unforgettable panic attack, I was still feeling on edge with free-floating anxiety. I went to a local gynecologist thinking it might be a hormonal imbalance due to perimenopause. This conventional doctor recommended a popular antidepressant and a Pap smear! I told her point-blank: "I'm not depressed—I'm just feeling overwhelmed."

Meanwhile, I did have my hormone levels checked upon *my* request. Plus, I sought a second opinion. Both the general practitioner and I agreed my anxiety was linked to stress. And when my test results came back, I knew that my hormones were not out of whack. The lesson: Go the extra mile to get a second opinion or get tests, or you may end up in a sequel to *One Flew over the Cuckoo's Nest!*

The advantage of going to a more experienced physician in the community, adds Dr. Thomas, is that they know most of the local doctors and will be able to recommend a good one if you need a specialist. However, for example, if a patient has an orthopedic problem there may be only one orthopedic surgeon available on their insurance list. But that doesn't have to be a problem.

"What the patient can do in that case is appeal to their insurance company, and they're mandated by law to go out of the plan to get a second opinion," points out Dr. Thomas. And it may be worth your while to do this, so you won't have to pay out of pocket.

Keep in mind that there are several routes to the healing process. If the second opinion differs from the first, you'll have to be the judge and decide which treatment is right for you.

In this book, you'll realize soon enough that not all of the 101 doctors agree with one another. In fact, I have included second opinions in some chapters. Once again, *you* will have to make the final decision regarding the right route to take for your wellbeing. And you'll discover that while these doctors don't always agree, they're on the same road to preventive good health and longevity.

HOW THIS BOOK CAN WORK FOR YOU AND YOUR FAMILY

Part I, "The Heart, Blood, and Brain," explains how important it is to stay heart-healthy no matter what your age or gender.

You'll learn why understanding the numbers of your cholesterol and blood pressure levels are important. And, better yet, you'll discover how diet, nutrients, herbs, and lifestyle changes can play a big role in heart health.

Part II, "Good Diet, Bad Absorption," will help you understand why it is necessary to have optimal digestion for overall good health. Solutions to common stomach problems will help you get a handle on keeping your digestive tract in order. It will give you step-by-step tips for both prevention and treatment of tummy troubles.

Part III, "From Colds to Cancer," discusses your built-in defense system. Once you learn why it's vital to keep your immunity strong, you'll be eager to use our doctors' dietary advice, tips, and supplement plans to help you stave off colds, flu, and even cancer.

Part IV, "Bones, Joints, and Muscles," discusses the importance of a healthy spine and bones. This section gives you details about all the ways doctors stave off aches and pains in themselves, family, and patients. And you will learn how diet, vitamins and minerals, and exercise play a big role in building and preserving healthy bones, joints, and muscles for both men and women at any age.

Part V, "All in the Head," gives you detailed instructions on how doctors keep their cool, whether it be anxiety, depression, or stress—or some combination of the three. This section gives you advice, tips, and techniques to use every day that will help you chill out from head to toe.

Part VI, "The Female Body," will help you understand how you can lower the risk of developing hormonal-related symptoms and disease. Women docs who've been there, done that will help you get a handle on what to expect and how to prevent problems only a woman can understand.

Part VII, "The Male Body," provides the lowdown on men's health problems from a male perspective. You'll learn how diet, supplements, and exercise have helped male doctors help themselves, family members, and patients. Their advice and inspirational stories will help you to make some changes that may help you live a longer and better life.

Part VIII, "Mind, Body and Spirit," includes a mega health list on how to keep your total body healthy. A variety of doctors will show you exactly how many factors, from your teeth and libido to environmental toxins and spirituality, can play a big role in your mind, body, and spirit.

MORE HEALING INFO

In addition, I provide you with some basic statistics (regarding major diseases and disorders), their risk factors, and the age and gender groups primarily affected. Extra facts for your information will be derived from doctors, surveys, or national health organizations. And, some of the medical words are easy enough to understand, but others need a human translation.

Keep in mind, preventive and treatable maladies can often manifest into out-of-control diseases. By using some physical checkup reminders, you'll be doing as the doctors do—practicing preventive care, which will help you to live a longer and healthier life.

Also, some of the doctors provide unforgettable anecdotes about patients that they have treated. These stories illustrate how diet, supplements, and lifestyle changes can and do make a difference in improving health.

Most important, you will find dozens of easy-to-read supplement charts showing the vitamins, minerals, and herbs that some of the 101 doctors interviewed take or recommend to their family and patients. You'll discover that some doctors note their personal or recommended dosages; other doctors omit the dosages because they vary for each individual. Please consult with your doctor regarding what doses are right for you.

Be sure to read the directions on the supplement label and consult with your doctor before starting any new vitamin, mineral, herb, or food supplement. You can also check out the "Safety Smarts" pointers throughout the book. But note, supplement precautions are controversial and vary from individual to individual.

Docs' Rx to Heal Yourself

- In this book, you'll learn the importance of good nutrition.
- In this book, you'll discover how vitamins, minerals, and herbs can help to supplement your diet for optimal health.
- In this book, you'll learn how to maintain your total body.
- In this book, you'll learn how an ounce of prevention can improve and even save your life.
- In this book, you'll learn how to live a longer and healthier life.
- In this book, you'll discover how using doctors' personal strategies can be one of the best things you can do for your health.

Bios

Earl Mindell, Ph.D., at 61, is a registered pharmacist, nutritionist, and master herbalist. He attended the College of Pharmacy of North Dakota State University and got his Ph.D. at Pacific Western in Los Angeles, California. He has written dozens of books including *Earl Mindell's Vitamin Bible for the 21st Century* (Time Warner). He currently writes and lectures. Web site: Healthvoyage. com. Product line: 888-345-6709; DrEarl.com. He is married, has two children, and resides in Beverly Hills, California.

Jack Thomas, D.O., is a 53-year-old internist and family practitioner who attended Philadelphia College of Osteopathic Medicine. He is program director of Family Practice Residency at Pacific Hospital in Long Beach, California, and also clinic director for the Pacific Family Health Clinic in Long Beach. He resides in Long Beach with his wife and two children.

PART I

The Heart, Blood, and Brain

Whenever I think of heart health, I get images of my late mom complaining about heart murmurs. For years I used to wonder if I had inherited her heart problems. But I wasn't sure. I do know that I have abstained from alcohol and cigarettes, and I stay active—unlike my mother. Getting physical—walking, swimming, and weight training—has been in my routine since childhood.

Mom's doctors had her taking blood pressure medication. But with the help of eating right and trying to chill out (that one is tough for me), I am keeping my blood pressure down naturally. (Yesterday it was 114/77.) And, so far, my heart is healthy as I inch toward the big 50.

Just like my mother, who eventually had a mini-stroke, many of you may not know all of the natural things that you can do to keep heart-healthy. The key to having a healthy heart is to follow a preventive heart-healthy game plan.

In Part I, "The Heart, Blood, and Brain," cardiologist Dr. Seth Baum, author of *The Total Guide to a Healthy Heart* (Kensington), says, "The heart is clearly the most important organ in the body. Preventive measures absolutely can help to prevent heart disease."

Christie Ballantyne, M.D., another heart doctor, explains what "good" and "bad" cholesterol means and why you should care about keeping your levels in check.

Dr. John McDougall, author of *The McDougall Program for a Healthy Heart* (Dutton), states, "Your primary approach is to take advantage of every benefit that comes from correcting your diet and lifestyle."

Dr. Stephen T. Sinatra, a cardiologist, declares, "The best approach to heart disease is marrying the conventional and the alternative approach; blend both camps together to give the patient the greatest arsenal in their battle against heart disease." And the other doctors in this section will tell you everything you want to know about the heart of the matter but were afraid to ask.

1

Angina

Dr. Baum's Heart-Healthy Plan

SETH BAUM, M.D.

I first heard of angina from one of my editors. He's not the typical Type A, driven, impatient personality. He's more of a Type B—easygoing and calm. But, he admits, he wasn't always like that.

At 43, this editor had angina (chest pain), a warning sign that the heart is being affected by lack of oxygen. During recovery from two angioplasty treatments, he revamped his lifestyle.

I turned to Dr. Seth Baum, a cardiologist, to discuss prevention of angina (also known as angina pectoris), which is just one of the many types of heart problems he sees daily. "Angina is a manifestation of coronary disease. So when people have coronary disease they often develop angina. It is the rare individual with coronary disease who does not have angina," he explains.

Common symptoms of angina are shortness of breath with exertion, fatigue with exercise, and belly pain. However, the typical place for the chest pain is under the breastbone a little to the left.

So how does Dr. Baum know if his patients have angina? "Angina is a symptom. The way you determine what a symptom is, is on the history. We listen to the patient, we ask questions, and we try to discern if they're having angina," he explains. Once Dr. Baum discovers his patients have angina, what is his heart-healthy game plan?

"It depends on the patient. It depends on how rapidly the angina occurred. I put all patients—with angina and without angina—on an improved diet (low-fat, low-cholesterol), an exercise regimen, and stress reduction techniques," says Dr. Baum.

"What is very important is stress reduction. But you have to distinguish between angina and coronary disease. Angina means that you're having pain from coronary disease," points out Dr. Baum. Simply put, if you have chest pain it's your body telling you that you need to fight heart disease, and the goal is to limit risk factors by practicing the following preventive measures.

FACTS F.Y.I.

According to the Amercian Heart Association:

- About 400,000 new cases of stable angina (predictable chest pain on exertion or under mental or emotional stress) and about 150,000 new cases of unstable angina (unexpected chest pain while at rest) occur each year.
- Approximately 27 percent of men and 14 percent of women will develop angina within six years after a recognized heart attack.
- Only 20 percent of coronary attacks are preceded by long-standing angina.

FIVE HEART-TO-HEART TIPS

These tips are from Dr. Baum:

- *Eat a low-fat, low-cholesterol diet.* By eating a healthful diet you can lower your blood pressure and cholesterol levels, which can help reduce angina symptoms.

- *Learn how to cope with stress by using destressing techniques.* Angina is usually caused by a lack of blood supply and oxygen to the cells of your heart muscle, which can occur after an emotional upset. It can be relieved by rest and relaxation.
- *Don't smoke.* It constricts blood vessels. It makes platelets more active, so they're more sticky and your blood is more likely to clot.
- *Enjoy some wine.* Alcohol can be beneficial in moderation, especially red wine. It's not just the disease-fighting antioxidant effect, it can raise the HDL levels (high-density lipoprotein, the "good" cholesterol), too.
- *Get a move on.* Keeping physical on a regular basis can help you stay slim and fit, which can help you lower your blood pressure and cholesterol, which are also a part of lessening angina symptoms.

SUCCESS STORY

"Let me tell you about the first person I took through an integrative approach to heart disease," Dr. Baum says. "One man, at 60, came to me and had an abnormal stress test. He had just recently developed angina. He had angina attacks whenever he played tennis. So I did an angiogram (an X-ray of the blood vessels to diagnose heart problems) on him and saw his arteries, which had significant blockages. I recommended a bypass (in which veins or arteries from the leg are placed to bypass the blockages in the arteries that feed the heart).

"But after I walked out of the room I thought, maybe this is somebody I can take a different approach with. The next day I offered him an alternative approach, which included exercise, stress reduction, and nutritional supplements. He opted for that," recalls Dr. Baum.

The outcome: The man's stress test has since become normal. His angina is yesterday's news. And his cholesterol and blood pressure levels are in check. "It made me feel wonderful," says

Dr. Baum, "because I was able to help him avoid having a bypass operation, which would have been a traumatic and potentially life-threatening event."

THE DOC'S SUPPLEMENT LIST

These two heart-healthy nutrients are recommended by Dr. Baum to patients with heart disease and can help prevent and treat angina.

Supplement	What It Does
CoQ_{10}	This fat-soluble compound (also called coenzyme Q_{10}) acts as an antioxidant, improving the body's ability to use oxygen; it reduces symptoms of angina
Magnesium	This mineral helps your muscles relax and can lessen stress on the heart muscle; it can alleviate chest pain

DOC'S RX TO HEAL YOURSELF

- Get a heart checkup.
- Consume a low-fat, low-cholesterol diet.
- Opt for heart-healthy supplements such as magnesium and CoQ_{10}.
- Use destressing techniques.
- Avoid smoking, which can cause your blood to clot.
- Exercise regularly to prevent stress and emotional upsets.

Bio

Seth Baum, M.D., is a cardiologist at Integrative Heart Care in Boca Raton, Florida. He received his doctor of medicine degree from Columbia College in New York. He is the author of *The Total Guide to a Healthy Heart* (Kensington). At 41, he is married with three children and lives in Boca Raton.

2

Cholesterol Problems

DR. BALLANTYNE'S CHOLESTEROL CONTROLLERS

CHRISTIE BALLANTYNE, M.D.

Dr. Christie Ballantyne, a no-nonsense cardiologist, told me that the first step in lowering high cholesterol is to look at an individual's risk for heart disease. To do that means starting off with a set of questions about age and gender, which Dr. Ballantyne discusses in our interview about how he helps his patients and himself to control cholesterol, a fatty substance in the bloodstream.

Dr. Ballantyne explains that the older you get, the more your risk of high cholesterol goes up, for both men and women (for men it starts earlier than for women). Men, in addition to having high cholesterol levels, may have more problems with low levels of the high-density lipoprotein or HDL cholesterol, the "good" cholesterol that carries extra "bad" cholesterol and fat away. And men frequently have higher triglycerides (the stuff that causes your blood to clot, which can trigger a heart attack) than women.

On the flip side, women may have high levels of total cholesterol; however, a woman often has more of the good HDL cholesterol than the low-density lipoprotein or LDL cholesterol, the artery-clogging "bad" cholesterol. But the catch is, HDL drops during the menopausal years and LDL goes up.

Also important is the genetic factor: Do you know what your family history is (both parents and siblings) with premature heart disease? Plus, despite your genes playing a role in cholesterol levels, a big cause of low HDL is cigarette smoking, so smoking is an issue, too. The bottom line: It's important to know your cholesterol levels—HDL, LDL, and triglycerides.

PHYSICAL CHECKUP

Dr. Ballantyne and the American Heart Association (AHA) recommend that every adult have a lipid profile, which will calculate your total cholesterol and triglyceride levels. In adults, total cholesterol levels of 240 milligrams per deciliter (mg/dL) or higher are considered high risk, and levels from 200 to 239 mg/dL are considered borderline high risk. Also, it's a good idea to get a glucose test and a urine test to detect any other potential factors that can cause a lipid problem.

GETTING THE ODDS IN YOUR FAVOR

According to Dr. Ballantyne, the ideal would be an HDL cholesterol level of over 40, an LDL cholesterol level of less than 100, and a triglyceride level of less than 150.

Once you know what your personal risk factors are, there are things you can do to lower your cholesterol and triglyceride levels to reduce your risk from heart disease, says Dr. Ballantyne.

- *Diet.* Dr. Ballantyne recommends a diet that is low in saturated fat and low in cholesterol. The problem is, when you read labels and the products say "low-fat, low-cholesterol," it's a calorie trap. The manufacturers just switch sugar for fat. Therefore, people tend to gain weight, which can play a role in cholesterol levels.

- *More Protein Please.* "Some people do a little better with weight loss with a higher-protein diet. There's some controversy on optimal diet. If someone has a pure high cholesterol and they have normal triglyceride and a good HDL cholesterol, then diets that are very low in fat and very low in cholesterol—like the Dean Ornish diet (a vegetarian diet of less than 10 percent calories in fat and zero cholesterol)—work very well," explains Dr. Ballantyne.

  On the other hand, a higher-protein diet may be the key to weight loss for other folks, says Dr. Ballantyne. For a lot of people their problem ends up being more of a triglyceride and HDL problem—and they're overweight. For these people, the real key is weight loss.

  "We say you need to focus on your sugars, you're taking in too many carbohydrates, saturated fats are bad but some of the monounsaturated fats are better. For example, fish oils—omega-3 and omega-6 essential fatty acids—have some protective effects for cardiovascular disease. We shift them sometimes to a higher-protein diet. Some of these people get a lean cut of meat that is low in fat, and that is actually far healthier than eating a whole bunch of carbos. And it may give them more satiety to help them lose weight," explains Dr. Ballantyne.

- *Exercise.* It is believed that regular exercise can raise the good HDL. Dr. Ballantyne likes to set a specific regular program. He encourages people to join a gym and work out or get a personal trainer.

- *The Medical Option.* If high cholesterol is not responding to these preventive strategies, or if a patient has many risk factors, Dr. Ballantyne says he starts them on medications. "The best medicines for high cholesterol are the statins such as Lipitor, which lowers your bad LDL cholesterol, also lowers the triglycerides, and raises the good HDL levels," he says.

- *One Baby Aspirin a Day.* Also, if you have high cholesterol, it's more of a reason to take a baby aspirin each day.

Remember, what causes a heart attack is not just the buildup of a blockage but the blood clot on the blockage.

- *B Vitamins.* Folic acid, B_6, and B_{12} for reducing homocysteine (an amino acid), another risk factor, may help keep your cholesterol levels in check. "We don't have any evidence that lowering homocysteine reduces heart attacks, but studies are in progress, and it's not unreasonable to take B complex vitamins," he says.

TAKING CARE OF HIS OWN CHOLESTEROL LEVELS

Meanwhile, as Dr. Ballantyne treats his patients with the above strategies, what about his own cholesterol levels? "I have a bad family history. My father had a heart attack when he was 55," he points out.

Two heart scans showed that Dr. Ballantyne had some calcium in his arteries (some blockage) so he is getting his LDL to less than 100 by taking a cholesterol-lowering drug.

Plus, he watches his diet and exercises. "My HDL has always been above 40; my triglycerides are below 150; my LDL is about 135 to 145. My thought is, because of some genetic susceptibility I probably have to maintain a very low LDL cholesterol."

THE DOC'S SUPPLEMENT LIST

Here are some of the supplements Dr. Ballantyne recommends to his patients to win the cholesterol number game.

Supplement	What It Does
Folic Acid, B_6, and B_{12}	These B vitamins can help lower homocysteine in your body, which may help you keep your cholesterol levels in check.

| Omega-3s and omega-6s | These essential fatty acids have protective effects for heart disease. |
| Baby aspirin | Can help prevent blood clotting. |

Safety Smarts: Omega oils: Don't take high doses of fish oil capsules if you are taking NSAIDs (nonsteroidal anti-inflammatory drugs). It may increase gastrointestinal ulcers and bleeding.

DOC'S RX TO HEAL YOURSELF

- Eat a low-fat, low-cholesterol diet to keep your cholesterol levels healthy.
- If you are overweight, lose weight to keep your "good" HDL cholesterol levels up.
- Opt for more protein in your diet if your triglycerides and HDL cholesterol numbers are a problem.
- Take omega-3s and omega-6s to protect against heart disease.
- Don't forget your B vitamins—folic acid, B_6, and B_{12}—to keep homocysteine levels down and cholesterol levels normal.

BIO

Christie Ballantyne, M.D., went to medical school at Baylor College of Medicine in Houston, Texas. He is director of the Center of Cardiovascular Prevention at Methodist Debakey Heart Center in Houston and professor of medicine at Baylor College of Medicine. At 45, he is married, has three children, and resides in Houston. Web site: www.lipidsonline.org.

3

Heart Disease

Dr. McDougall's Lifesaving Diet

JOHN MCDOUGALL, M.D.

When I wrote a weekly diet and nutrition column for *Woman's World*, I often interviewed the diet guru Dr. John McDougall about dietary fiber and health. I was always amazed and impressed that the doctor himself ate 60 to 100 grams of fiber daily.

As we reconnected, he told me that he weighs 173 pounds and is six foot one inch tall. Even more inspiring is that Dr. McDougall is now in his fifties and adds that he windsurfs. So I got the picture fast. He is still the epitome of health.

According to Dr. McDougall, "Heart disease and strokes are not due to any deficiency in aspirin or fish oil. The wisest way to prevent tragedies from a defective blood vessel system is to deal with the cause: Your first-line therapy should be a low-fat, no-cholesterol diet." And Dr. McDougall follows this type of diet plan to a *T* (except on special occasions such as Thanksgiving and fishing trips).

"I eat well," he quips. "I get people all of the time who tell me they eat 'well.' They eat chicken, fish, and low-fat milk. But that's not quite going to do it. You really have to cut these things completely to get the kind of health that I would like to have. And so I eat a pure vegetarian diet," he says.

"If you want to prevent heart disease, you want to eat a plant-based diet. There is no cholesterol and it's high in vegetable protein—it has no animal protein or saturated fat. The diet avoids artery-damaging fat and cholesterol and provides health-promoting antioxidants and other phytochemicals," explains Dr. McDougall. And this healthful type of nutrient-dense diet is key to prevention of heart disease.

He adds, "I don't prescribe aspirin for anybody unless they've had a heart attack, bypass surgery, or angioplasty. If that's the case, then I do prescribe it. But if you haven't had that history then you're at such low risk for heart disease that the adverse effects (such as gastrointestinal bleeding) of the aspirin outweigh the benefits."

Unlike the majority of the 101 doctors interviewed in this book, Dr. McDougall does not take supplements for heart disease prevention. He relies on a sensible diet, daily exercise, and healthy habits.

FACT F.Y.I.

According to the American Heart Association:

• Heart disease is the number-one killer of American men and women in the United States.

THE DOC'S HEART-SMART FAVORITE FOODS

Burritos
Chili with rice
Hash brown potatoes
Mu shu vegetables

Oatmeal
Pancakes
Spaghetti
Vegetable soups
Veggie sandwiches and burgers
Waffles

SECOND OPINION: COMBINATION THERAPY WITH DR. JANSON

MICHAEL JANSON, M.D.

Dr. Michael Janson is another doctor who practices what he preaches. A medical doctor who specializes in preventive nutrition, he has both a personal and a professional interest in heart health.

At 18 he was diagnosed with a leaky heart valve, a condition that can lead to the heart's inability to cope with the amount of blood it needs to pump. The doctors predicted that within 20 or 30 years he would have congestive heart failure. But it didn't happen.

Meanwhile, he is healthy, and he takes heart-healthy supplements that he recommends to his patients with heart problems (such as high blood pressure, heart attack recovery, high cholesterol, and stroke prevention). And this is no surprise since he is the author of *Dr. Janson's New Vitamin Revolution* (Penguin USA).

"Most of us have seen the benefits of supplements in practice," concludes Dr. Janson who is a devout advocate of nutrition and alternative medicine, like many of the other doctors in this book.

THE DOC'S SUPPLEMENT LIST

Here are six heart-healthy supplements that Dr. Janson recommends.

Supplement	What It Does
Magnesium	A heart-smart mineral that is used for high blood pressure. It relaxes muscles of blood vessels, which opens them up and lowers high blood pressure.
CoQ_{10}	It is a natural substance found in food important for lowering blood pressure; it is a fat-soluble antioxidant compound. It is a cofactor for the production of an energy molecule called ATP inside each cell. We make it in our own bodies, but we don't make enough as we age.
Hawthorn	It is an herb that helps to lower high blood pressure and prevent heart disease and heart attack. Dilates blood vessels; dilates coronary vessels and aids in blood supply to the heart, which reduces angina attacks; stabilizes cardiac activity and inhibits arrhythmias.
Garlic	It is an herb used for heart health. Inhibits LDL production; improves use of dietary cholesterol; lessens artery blockage; improves blood flow; a sulfur-containing compound called allicin helps lower cholesterol and blood pressure and prevents blood clots.
Arginine	It is an amino acid that is a blood vessel relaxant. It is a precursor to nitric oxide, a substance that also relaxes the blood vessels.

| Gamma-linolenic acid | It is an essential oil that your body needs to make certain regulatory substances that help reduce blood vessel spasms. It helps to open up blood vessels. |

Safety Smarts: Hawthorn: Consult with your doctor before using hawthorn, especially if you have low blood pressure. Garlic: Do not use garlic before surgery (it's a blood thinner). If you are already taking blood-thinning medicine or aspirin, consult with your doctor first.

Dr. Simopoulos's Omega Fats

ARTEMIS P. SIMOPOULOS, M.D.

While eating heart-healthy foods can certainly help to reduce your risk of heart disease, so can eating "good fats"—essential fatty acids. That's exactly what Dr. Artemis P. Simopoulos, author of *The Omega Diet* (HarperPerennial), will tell you.

Simply put, there are two kinds of essential fatty acids (EFAs), omega-6 and omega-3. The problem: The American diet contains more omega-6 fatty acids (found in foods such as mayonnaise and salad dressing) than omega-3s. This imbalance makes us more prone to heart disease, according to Dr. Simopoulos.

In other words, the good doctor says that we can eat foods that contain the "good" fats—eggs, fish, and even chocolate—and plenty of antioxidant-rich fruits, vegetables, and legumes. Eating these foods, as do heart-healthy people in the Mediterranean countries, can protect your cardiovascular system by raising your antioxidant levels, reducing your risk of blood clots, and aid in normalizing your blood pressure and heartbeat.

Omega-3 oils may raise HDL (good) cholesterol, lower or slightly increase LDL (bad) cholesterol, lower blood pressure, and lower risk of blood clots. That means a diet rich in omega-3 fatty acids can help fight against heart disease. In fact, research shows that a diet that is low in saturated fat, low in trans fatty acids, balanced in omeg-3 and omega-6, and rich in fruits and vegetables is heart-healthy. The following are tips from Dr. Simopoulos:

SEVEN DIETARY TIPS TO BALANCE THE EFAS IN YOUR DIET

- *Enrich your diet with omega-3 fatty acids.* Eat fatty fish two or more times a week (you could satisfy that requirement by eating two generous portions of salmon) or take omega-3 supplements.
- *Use canola oil or olive oil as your primary oil.* Canola oil provides monounsaturated fatty acids and LNA, the plant form of omega-3 fatty acids; olive oil has life-enhancing properties.
- *Eat seven or more servings of fruits and vegetables daily.* People in Mediterranean countries consume plenty of fresh produce and have enjoyed good health due to the antioxidant benefits.
- *Eat more peas, beans, and nuts.* They are free of saturated fat and cholesterol.
- *Eat less saturated fat and cholesterol.* Both of these increase the risk of heart disease.
- *Avoid oils high in omega-6 fatty acids.* These include corn oil, safflower oil, peanut oil, soybean oil, sunflower seed oil, cottonseed oil, mayonnaise, and salad dressing.
- *Avoid trans fatty acids.* If you see "partially hydrogenated" on a food label, forgo the product. These substances are often found in baked goods and snack foods.

THE DOC'S SUPPLEMENT LIST

Here is the number-one supplement that Dr. Simopoulos recommends.

Supplement	What It Does
Omega-3 fatty acids	Include more omega-3s in your diet to get the right balance of essential fatty acids in your diet

Safety Smarts: Omega-3 oils: Don't take high doses of fish oil capsules if you are taking NSAIDs (nonsteroidal anti-inflammatory drugs). It may increase gastrointestinal ulcers and bleeding.

DR. McCULLY'S VITAMIN B BREAKTHROUGH

KILMER S. McCULLY, M.D.

Truth is, I've never had my cholesterol levels checked. The good news is, having low cholesterol may not be the key to heart disease after all, according to Dr. Kilmer S. McCully, author of *The Homocysteine Revolution* (Keats) and coauthor of *The Heart Revolution* (HarperPerennial).

In his books and our interview he told me that I can cut my risk of heart disease by controlling the real enemy, homocysteine—a little amino acid. Thirty years ago he discovered that homocysteine has an important role in the underlying cause of arteriosclerosis (hardening of the arteries), blood pressure, stroke, and even heart attack.

He explains that if high levels of this substance build up in your bloodstream, due to a nutritional deficiency of three B vitamins—B_6, B_{12}, and folic acid—you will be more at risk for developing heart disease.

These three specific B vitamins are lacking in our Western diet.

"The reason the Mediterranean diet is beneficial is that the foods contain a higher amount of these three vitamins—B_6, folic acid, and B_{12}." The traditional Mediterranean diet contains an abundance of fresh vegetables, fresh fruits, fresh fish, fresh organ meats, and whole-grain products. People who eat the Mediterranean diet tend to have a lower level of homocysteine in the blood than those who eat a more Northern-style diet, explains Dr. McCully.

He adds, "The deficiency of these B vitamins is caused by food processing. The traditional methods of food processing like milling of grains and addition of chemical additives all lead to serious depletion of these B vitamins from the foods."

Dr. McCully recommends these six dietary tips to help you start eating a more heart-healthy and vitamin B–rich diet:

- Eat more fresh vegetables and fruits daily to get enough folic acid, vitamin B_6, and other beneficial nutrients.
- Avoid canned vegetables; the heat of processing can destroy up to 80 percent of the vitamin B_6 and folic acid.
- Steam vegetables in a limited amount of water to keep the B vitamins in.
- Eat whole-wheat cereal, brown rice, and root vegetables. Eliminate white rice, white flour, and refined sugar.
- Eat one to two servings of fresh fish, meat, or eggs per day.
- A couple of times a month, eat liver, a rich source of vitamin B_6, vitamin B_{12}, and folic acid, since, according to Dr. McCully, "a multivitamin may not contain enough of B_6, B_{12}, and folic acid to reduce homocysteine to the desirable level." One-third fat, one-third protein, and one-third natural carbohydrates is the right balance.

So does Dr. McCully practice what he preaches? "My wife and I have eaten this diet for many years. We have tried to improve our diet as the knowledge about it improves. We have really eaten the diet described in *The Heart Revolution*. We follow the diet quite closely and we're both healthy," he told me.

These days, however, Dr. McCully is taking supplements.

"The reason is that measuring my blood homocysteine level five years ago revealed a slightly elevated level. Before starting *The Heart Revolution Diet,* my level was 10.6 micromoles per liter. After I had been eating this diet for three years and taking small amounts of B_6, B_{12}, and folic acid, the level had fallen to 7.3! Recently, however, at the age of 67, my level has increased to 11.3, probably because of the aging process."

He adds, "Populations with homocysteine levels of 6 to 8 have significantly less heart disease than populations with 10 to 12 micromoles per liter. I have not yet measured my level after this increase in B vitamin supplements. So far I have no signs or symptoms of heart disease or other disease. I attribute my good health at present to *The Heart Revolution Diet* and to the beneficial genes that I inherited from my parents."

If you're wondering where you can go to get your own homocysteine level checked, "any commercial clinical laboratory or large medical center clinical laboratory can do homocysteine analysis of a fasting blood sample, when sent by your physician," says Dr. McCully.

THE DOC'S SUPPLEMENT LIST

Here are the B vitamins and other supplements that Dr. McCully is currently taking in an effort to reduce his homocysteine level to the desirable level of less than 8.0 micromoles per liter.

Supplement	What It Does	Dose
Multivitamin	Contains 3 mg B_6, which is sufficient to reduce homocysteine	One a day
Vitamin B_{12}	Reduces homocysteine level	250 mcg
Vitamin E	Reduces homocysteine level	400 IU
Folic acid	This B vitamin controls homocysteine	800 mcg

DR. GOULSTON'S TYPE A-B PERSONALITY QUIZ

MARK GOULSTON, M.D.

Did you know that certain personality types may be unhealthy for you and your lifestyle? There are two basic personality types, and based on your answers, psychiatrist Dr. Mark Goulston will tell you what kind of personality behavior is right for both you and your mate. Plus, he'll provide tips on how to cope better with unhealthy behavioral traits for your heart's sake.

1. Does a weekend with your mate include movies, shopping, and errands because you have to do it all?

    Yes   No

2. Is it important that you make it to the top of your dog-eat-dog workplace, even if you have to claw your way there?

    Yes   No

3. Are you often discontented with your or your mate's achievements?

    Yes   No

4. Is it difficult to say "I love you?"

    Yes   No

5. Do you feel anxiety before and during lovemaking?

    Yes   No

6. Do you find yourself honking in traffic even though you know your impatience irks your partner?

    Yes   No

7. Do you feel that you have to be a better lover than your mate's past lovers?

    Yes   No

8. Would you rather work more and make more

money than talk about your feelings with
you-know-who?   Yes   No

9. Is your favorite pastime acquiring worldly
   possessions for both you and your true love?   Yes   No

10. Do you find it hard to sit and do nothing with
    (or without) your significant other?   Yes   No

How Did You Score?

Tally up your answers (the number of yes's and no's) to find
out your personality type—Type A (first studied by heart specialist Dr. Meyer Friedman) or Type B (defined as the lack of Type A
behavior).

Mostly Yes

Type A: You have a compulsion to win. Getting irritated or
easily angered is part of your nature. And waiting in lines is not
for you—no way! It can make your blood pressure soar. You eat,
walk and talk fast. After all, you have people to meet, places to
go. That means you are a demanding, high-powered go-getter
(which can raise your risk of heart disease).

Mostly No

Type B: You are more calm and less hurried than Type A. It's
difficult for you to do two things at a time—but then, why would
you want to? Warm and friendly, you love to listen to your mate
talk—unlike Type A's, who always interrupt. And you are likely
to enjoy yourself on vacation, even if your partner has to foot the
bill! The good news is, all of this laid-back behavior is heart-
healthy.

What Your Answers Mean

Once you understand your personality type, you can use this
knowledge to understand your mate (or select a mate) who is

compatible with you. This, in turn, will enhance your relationship (long-standing or new), and you'll both be healthier and happier.

Dr. Goulston, author of *The 6 Secrets of a Lasting Relationship: How to Fall in Love Again—and Stay There* (Putnam), provides the anxiety-provoking pros and cons of four personality combinations:

- *A+A.* With two superachiever Type A's, you'll have somebody who'll understand your expectations and not try to slow you down. They'll get the world that you live in. The downside is that while you're on the same wavelength, you'll be arguing about who pays attention to whom.
- *A+B.* For the Type A woman, a Type B man will be flexible and not critical of you. However, you may find yourself critical of him because you would like him to be more ambitious.
- *B+B.* If you're both B's, you'll find life is less chaotic for you. You'll be able to smell the roses and not get trampled in the race of life. The downside is that if you change your mind and want some of those material comforts, you may not get them if you're with another B.
- *B+A.* If you're a Type B woman and he's a Type A man, you'll get a take-charge guy who'll stand up for you and himself against the world. You'll feel protected. But you may feel inferior to him, because he'll be more ambitious.

COPING WITH TYPE A UNHEALTHY BEHAVIOR

According to Dr. Goulston, high-energy, goal-oriented Type A people (such as many of our 101 doctors) can be prone to stress, which can play a role in increasing their risk of developing hypertension, heart disease, colds, and even cancer.

Dr. Goulston (a self-professed Type A-B combo) says his Type A behavior comes out when he is writing books and lecturing. When he listens to his patients and at home, the Type B behavior is put to use. Dr. Goulston recommends these five easy alterations in your daily life. They'll help you to chill out and improve your heart health day to day:

- *Learn to say no.* Dr. Goulston recommends this strategy for peace of mind. On a card, write: "It's better to decline a potential high-stress event or situation rather than have regrets later." (Keep that just-say-no card by the telephone or calendar!)
- *Think before you react.* Before reacting to a high-stress situation, try to understand it first. "Counting to ten before you react can enable you to respond more effectively," says Dr. Goulston.
- *Talk to a friend.* Often, Type A people feel isolated in their troubles, which can intensify stress. But when you talk to a friend, it stops the aloneness, explains Dr. Goulston.
- *Hug a dog or cat.* Pets are ready-made stress reducers, and past research shows that pets can help reduce high blood pressure, a symptom often experienced by Type As. "Pets don't make demands of us," says Dr. Goulston, "so we're getting an unconditional show of affection, acknowledgment, and warmth."
- *Take control.* "Part of the evidence that you're healthy comes when you get into situations that used to stress you out and make you do unhealthy behaviors," points out Dr. Goulston. Rather than getting upset fast and turning to bad behavior, like a typical Type-A individual, you deal with the situation.

DOCS' RX TO HEAL YOURSELF

- Eat a plant-based diet to prevent heart disease.
- Take heart-healthy supplements—magnesium, CoQ_{10}, hawthorn, garlic, gamma-linolenic acid (GLA)—to keep your cholesterol and blood pressure levels low, improve blood flow, and inhibit clots.

- Balance your ratio of essential fatty acids—omega-3s and omega-6s—to restore your body's healthful nutritional balance.
- If you're not getting enough B vitamins in your diet—B_6, B_{12}, and folic acid—opt for supplements to lower your homocysteine level.
- Learn healthy strategies to modify your Type A behavior or to understand a Type A individual's behavior better, which will lower your risk of developing heart disease.

Bios

Mark Goulston, M.D., is an assistant clinical professor of psychiatry at the University of California at Los Angeles and a Fellow of the American Psychiatric Association. A graduate of Boston University Medical School, he did his psychiatric training at UCLA. He is coauthor of *Get Out of Your Own Way: Overcoming Self-Defeating Behavior* (Perigee Books). He maintains a private practice in Santa Monica, California, where he specializes in seeing couples and families. He lives in Los Angeles with his wife and three children.

Michael Janson, M.D., is a 56-year-old medical doctor who specializes in nutrition and preventive medicine and practices in Arlington, Massachusetts. He went to Boston University School of Medicine. He enjoys making pottery and gardening. Web site: www.drjanson.com. His *Healthy Living Newsletter* is available by e-mail or through QCI Nutritionals 1-888-922-4848 or www.qcinutritionals.com.

Kilmer S. McCully, M.D., is board certified by the American Board of Pathology in Anatomic and Clinical Pathology. He received his medical degree from Harvard Medical School in Boston, Massachusetts. In addition to being chief of pathology and laboratory medicine service at the West Roxbury VA Medical Center, he is also director of the Boston Area Consolidated

Laboratories for the Department of Veterans Affairs. In these positions he is a full-time employee of the federal government. At 67, he lives in Winchester, Massachusetts, is married, and has two children and two grandchildren.

John McDougall, M.D., is a board-certified internist. He attended Michigan State University. Dr. McDougall is the founder of the McDougall Wellness Clinic in Santa Rosa, California, and the McDougall Program at St. Helena Hospital in the Napa Valley, 1-800-358-9195. At 54, he resides in Santa Rosa, California. He is married and has three children. He is the author of several books including *The McDougall Program for Women* (Plume), which can be ordered at 1-800-570-1654. Web site: http://www.drmcdougall.com; to order Dr. McDougall's Right Foods call 1-800-367-3844.

Artemis P. Simopoulos, M.D., is president and founder of the Center for Genetics, Nutrition and Health, a nonprofit organization in Washington, D.C. She received her M.D. from Boston University School of Medicine and is a physician and endocrinologist whose research at the National Institutes of Health (NIH) was on the nutritional aspects of genetic and endocrine disorders.

4

High Blood Pressure

LOWER THE NUMBERS WITH DR. KENNEY'S PLAN

JAMES JAY KENNEY, PH.D.

Surprise! Destressing isn't the only thing you can do to prevent or control high blood pressure. By the time they reach their sixties, more than half of Americans, men and women, will have high blood pressure. The reason: too much salt, according to Dr. James Jay Kenney.

"I developed hypertension in my mid-twenties. It rose above 140/90 [considered high blood pressure; 120/80 is optimal]. By the time I was in my early thirties it was about 150/100. It was high because I ate too much salty food," Dr. Kenney told me.

"Once you develop a condition, you become much more interested in research related to that condition. I started reading literature about salt and hypertension. It didn't take long to figure out that salt was the primary culprit," he recalls. So he lowered his sodium intake and lowered his blood pressure, too.

Today, Dr. Kenney proudly reveals that his blood pressure is very low—100/60. "It's downright un-American," he laughs. "You tend not to see blood pressures that low in otherwise healthy people who are eating typical Westernized diets with a lot of processed foods."

Dr. Kenney adds, "The lower your blood pressure is over time, the longer you're likely to live." That's because you'll be less likely to have a stroke or heart attack. No doubt the doctor is happy that his blood pressure is low these days. However, he pays the price because his diet is bland. After all, he knows and I know that low-sodium foods exclude pizza, store-bought spaghetti sauce, and television dinners—the convenient, fun fare.

"I don't eat much salt. Scientific research proves that a low-salt diet lowers blood pressure in people who have normal blood pressure. It lowers it even more in people that have high blood pressure."

FACTS F.Y.I.

According to the American Heart Association:

- Nearly 50 million Americans have high blood pressure, also called hypertension.
- An estimated one in four adults have high blood pressure; however, about 30 percent don't know they have it.

DOCTORS' LINGO

Blood Pressure: Blood pressure consists of two forces: the power the heart exerts each time it pumps blood and the resistant force the walls of the arteries exert against this push. Blood pressure is shown as two readings: the top number is the systolic pressure, which describes the heart's force; the bottom number is the diastolic pressure, the tension between heartbeats. (Definition courtesy of Cal Orey, "Drop That Blood Pressure," *Energy Times*, February 2001, page 38.)

SHAKE THE SODIUM HABIT

It's not enough to throw out the salt shaker. Most of the sodium Americans get comes from processed foods. That's why Dr. Kenney eats a very natural diet and recommends that you do the same. Here are some of the doctor's "Say No to Salt" tips:

- *Check food labels for sodium and calorie content.* Ideally the sodium level in the food you eat should average about half of your daily calorie intake. So if you're eating 2,400 calories a day, you should get 1,200 milligrams of sodium.
- *Avoid foods that have added salt.* Stay clear of foods in which the sodium level is higher than the calorie level per serving.
- *Cut down on processed foods.* Cheese, lunch meats and snack foods, canned soups and vegetables, and canned vegetable juice are very high in sodium.
- *Limit your intake of sodium to 1,500 milligrams or less a day.* This ensures maximum blood pressure reduction.

SAMPLE ONE-DAY LOW-SODIUM DIET PLAN

Breakfast: Whole-grain cereal with no added salt such as oatmeal or shredded wheat with bran, fruit, and nonfat milk.

Lunch: Whole-grain pasta with homemade marinara sauce made with tomato puree and canned tomatoes without added salt. (Store brands of marinara sauce are high in sodium. Dr. Kenney also adds heart-healthy olive oil, onion, garlic, and Italian blend seasoning.) Salad with homemade salad dressing made with canola oil, orange juice, or table wine. (Cooking wine usually contains salt.)

Snack: Unsalted nuts or fruit.

Dinner: Poached salmon. Brown rice. Steamed vegetables or salad.

Snack: Fresh fruit or soy ice cream.

RESEARCH IN A NUTSHELL

Without doubt, Dr. Kenney's low-sodium diet is in line with research at Johns Hopkins. This research confirmed that the Dietary Approaches to Stop Hypertension (DASH) diet, which is low in fat and high in fruits and vegetables and cuts back on fatty meats, lowers blood levels of homocysteine, an amino acid that circulates throughout the body and may raise the risk of heart disease. Lowering homocysteine by increasing your vegetable intake may lower your risk of developing high blood pressure. (Taking B vitamins may also lower homocysteine.)

HIGH BLOOD PRESSURE QUIZ

High blood pressure often can be controlled, especially for people with borderline (high normal) blood pressure. Take the following quiz to determine if you are at high risk:

1. Are you over the age of 65?   Yes   No
2. Do you have a family history of high blood
   pressure?   Yes   No
3. Are you postmenopausal?   Yes   No
4. Are you African-American?   Yes   No
5. Are you overweight and a sofa spud?   Yes   No
6. Do you sprinkle several teaspoons of salt on
   your meals?   Yes   No
7. Do you calm your frazzled nerves with more than
   two drinks per day?   Yes   No
8. Do you smoke?   Yes   No

9. Does your prescription for birth control include
   oral contraceptives?   Yes No
10. Do you feel stressed out 24/7?   Yes No

The more yes answers you gave, the more apt you are to be at
risk for high blood pressure. According to research, each of these
lifestyle choices can raise your blood pressure.

SECOND OPINION: DR. EDWARDS'S HERBAL REMEDIES

DAVID EDWARDS, M.D.

Dr. David Edwards is an internist with an interest in homeopathy and herbal medicine who helps people lower their blood
pressure. Interestingly, he told me that acupuncture can be used
in conjuction with blood pressure medication. "Some patients
that come in will be on blood pressure medicines," he points out.
"No one has talked to them about alternatives. They're either
getting side effects, or the costs are killing them, or they're very
suspicious that the drug may have some long-term effect that
they're not being told about."

First, he will find out if there is an underlying cause for high
blood pressure such as a weight problem. If so, he'll treat that
first and try to get the blood pressure down without treating the
pressure directly. Then, he may turn to acupuncture treatment,
which he was eager to discuss.

How does acupuncture work to help lower blood pressure?
"Endorphins are natural opiates in the brain that release under
certain stimuli, including acupuncture, that calm the conscious
and vegetative [blood pressure] systems down, relieving stress
and pain," explains Dr. Edwards.

For patients with high blood pressure he recommends acupuncture treatments as various circuits (pathways in the body)
are explored for clinical effect, he adds. "These usually include

the liver [Chinese theory of high blood pressure is "liver wind"] and the triple warmer-heart master circuits. These are said in Chinese theory to have function and constitute what the West would call the sympathetic [adrenaline] and parasympathetic [acetylcholine] neurotransmitter system. Sometimes, the heart-kidney acupuncture axis has to be used. The reasons are the same as in Western theory of high blood pressure."

For high blood pressure, acupuncture treatments are recommended twice a week for two to three weeks then begin spreading out to once a week until it's every three to four months, usually at the change of the seasons. Sessions last 15 to 25 minutes, depending on response. Effectiveness rate is about 20 to 25 percent depending on the individual's willingness and understanding of how it works. It also depends on the level of blood pressure and how long it's been there.

Docs' Rx to Heal Yourself

- Watch your sodium intake to drop that blood pressure.
- Eat more potassium-rich low-fat fruits and vegetables, which can deflate hypertension.
- Exercise can help lower your blood pressure.
- Destress yourself and watch those numbers plummet fast.
- Consider acupuncture treatments to help bring blood pressure down.

Bios

David Edwards, M.D., is a board-certified internist who received his M.D. at Creighton University School of Medicine in Omaha, Nebraska. He is also licensed in homeopathy and trained in acupuncture. He has a practice in Reno, Nevada, where he resides. At 56, he has three children.

James Jay Kenney, Ph.D., is board certified as an expert in human nutrition sciences by the American Board of Nutrition. He received his Ph.D. in nutrition from Rutgers University and is the nutrition research specialist at the Pritikin Longevity Center in Aventura, Florida. Web site: Foodandhealth.com. He is married at 56, has one child, and resides in Aventura.

5

Stroke

DR. SINATRA'S ANTI-STROKE STEPS

STEPHEN T. SINATRA, M.D.

The author of *Heart Disease and Women* (Lifeline Press), Stephen T. Sinatra, M.D., a veteran cardiologist, told me that stroke is an important topic for both men and women.

So what causes a stroke, anyhow? "The same thing that causes a heart attack. It can be a narrowing of a blood vessel in the brain or a blood clot," explains Dr. Sinatra. And strokes don't occur just in seniors either, he adds. "In a young woman or young man, if the blood clots in a strategic area, like the brain or heart, you can have a stroke."

As we get older, however, we are more prone to have a stroke, points out Dr. Sinatra. "High blood pressure is a major risk factor for stroke—more for a stroke than a heart attack."

FACTS F.Y.I.

According to the American Heart Association:

- Stroke is the third largest cause of death.
- An estimated 600,000 people suffer a new or recurrent stroke annually.
- It is believed that stroke is more common in men than in women.
- More than 50 percent of stroke deaths happen in women.
- The warning signs of a stroke are sudden numbness or weakness of the face, arm, or leg (especially on just one side of the body), sudden confusion, sudden trouble speaking or understanding, sudden trouble walking, dizziness, and sudden trouble seeing out of one or both eyes.

SEVEN WAYS TO PREVENT A STROKE

Here are the things that Dr. Sinatra practices and preaches to prevent a stroke.

- *Keep your blood pressure down.* High blood pressure is a precursor to stroke. You can control hypertension in many ways: diet, supplements, and lifestyle changes. (For more information, see Chapter 4.)
- *Get essential fatty acids—such as omega-3s—to prevent plaque rupture.* This nutrient can aid in lowering blood pressure (both systolic and diastolic) and is found in certain fish, fish oils, and flaxseed. Not only do they help lower high blood pressure, these "good fats" help lower LDL "bad" cholesterol and triglycerides and reduce platelet stickiness.
- *Take your nutrients.* According to Dr. Sinatra, the way CoQ_{10} brings down blood pressure isn't fully known. However, the membrane-stabilizing and antioxidant properties of CoQ_{10} may aid in normalizing cell chemistry in blood chemistry.

Like CoQ_{10}, L-carnitine can also enhance energy on a cellular level, which can lower your blood pressure.

- *Keep your weight down.* "Losing even 10 percent of your body weight can have a significant effect on lowering your blood pressure," points out Dr. Sinatra.
- *Exercise regularly.* An easy way to stay physical on a regular basis, which will help you to maintain your weight, is to walk between one and two miles every day, says Dr. Sinatra.
- *Don't smoke.* "Hypertensive smokers are three times more likely than nonsmokers to suffer stroke," points out Dr. Sinatra. "Smoking constricts your blood vessels."
- *Own your anger.* Do not explode in a rage. "Unresolved anger, high-stress lifestyle, and 'workaholism' all can contribute to high blood pressure," says Dr. Sinatra, who recommends developing an emotional support system. "There are many techniques to achieve this, including mental imagery, meditation, prayer, and biofeedback."

THE DOC'S SUPPLEMENT LIST

These are some supplements Dr. Stephen Sinatra recommends for stroke prevention.

Supplement	What It Does
Omega-3 fatty acids	These essential fatty acids prevent plaque blockage
CoQ_{10}	Helps to normalize cell chemistry in the blood
L-carnitine	Enhances energy on a cellular level

Safety Smarts: Omega-3 oils: Don't take high doses of fish oil capsules if you are taking NSAIDs (nonsteroidal anti-inflammatory drugs). It may increase gastrointestinal ulcers and bleeding.

SECOND OPINION: DR. LAIBOW'S BRAIN-BASED BIOFEEDBACK

RIMA LAIBOW, M.D.

In 1984, as a consequence of high blood pressure and a difficult pregnancy, ten days before the birth of her son, Dr. Rima Laibow suffered a serious stroke. "For six months I could not make sense of letters and numbers so I could not read. For about three years, the left side of my face drooped, especially when I was tired. My speech was slurred and I often said the wrong word," recalls Dr. Laibow.

"With time, these effects lessened so that nearly no one knew that I had been brain injured. I knew, however. For example, my reading speed dropped and never returned to my normal level," she adds.

In 1991, Dr. Laibow learned about neurobiofeedback (NBF) and started doing it for herself as well as her patients. She completed enough sessions so that she no longer could detect any consequences of the stroke.

DOCTOR'S LINGO

Neurobiofeedback: This treatment feeds the brain data it needs about the speed and efficiency with which neurons are communicating with one another. Each time a neuron communicates with others, an electrochemical pulse is released that produces the characteristic electrical activity that we read as the EEG (electroencephalogram).

An EEG is the summation of many frequencies passed through a computer, which separates out the individual frequencies of the brain activity. We have previously determined what the brain is doing compared to what it should be doing, so, with the frequency information that the computer provides, we can give the brain pleasant signals (light or sound) when it is acting in a normal way. The brain, to get more of these "reward signals," figures out how to do that. This, in turn, creates or reawakens necessary neural pathways.

NBF is an excellent preventive since high blood pressure, addictions to alcohol and cigarettes, and prolonged stress are known risk factors for cardiovascular diseases and stroke.

BIOFEEDBACK MAKES A COMEBACK

In 1999, Dr. Laibow had a ski injury that tore her retina. She turned to the techniques she had learned in NBF to heal her retina, since once a brain learns these skills, like writing or speaking, they are available when called upon.

Once home, she had medical tests, which documented the retinal injury, and an MRI (magnetic resonance imaging) to see what other damage had occurred. "Because the neurologist and radiologist knew my history they were astonished when they looked at my MRI, since not only was there no evidence of the retinal tear, but there was no longer any evidence that the brain we were looking at together had ever had a stroke."

In conclusion, Dr. Laibow learned that by doing NBF she was able to heal, at both the physical and the functional level, two serious injuries.

DOCS' RX TO HEAL YOURSELF

- Try supplements, less sodium, more fruits and vegetables, exercise, and destressing techniques to keep your blood pressure normal.
- Provide your body with the essential fatty acids it needs for cardiovascular health.
- Take supplements such as CoQ_{10} to keep your blood pressure down and L-carnitine to keep your healthy blood cells up.
- Healthy up your lifestyle by watching your weight, quitting smoking, and controlling your anger.

- Consider biofeedback to help prevent high blood pressure, addictions, and stress.

BIOS

Rima Laibow, M.D., is an integrative medicine psychiatrist in Croton on Hudson, New York. She attended Albert Einstein College of Medicine. She is 57 and works with her husband practicing neurobiofeedback, chelation, nutrition, meditation, stress management, and more. She has one son and resides in Croton on Hudson. For more information go to the web site www. drlaibow.com.

Stephen T. Sinatra, M.D., is a board-certified cardiologist and certified anti-aging specialist. He attended Albany Medical College and has more than 20 years of experience in helping patients prevent and reverse heart disease through integration of conventional medicine and complementary nutritional and psychological therapies. A Fellow in the American College of Cardiology, Dr. Sinatra is the author of *The Coenzyme Q_{10} Phenomenon* (Keats Publishing) and the editor of the monthly newsletter *Stephen Sinatra—The Sinatra Health Report* (formerly *Heart-Sense*)/*Advanced Biosolutions* (www.phillips.com/health/catalog .htm). Both his medical practice and home are in Manchester, Connecticut. He is married and has six children.

PART II

Good Diet, Bad Absorption

Ever hear "You are what you eat?" Truth is, you aren't that burger you ate for lunch but rather what you digest. I recently learned that even if you eat right, you still may not be getting enough vitamins and minerals from your food. That food must be broken down in the digestive tract, and the nutrients must be moved to the body's organs to be absorbed and utilized. And if you suffer common digestive complaints, you may not be digesting your food as well as you think.

In Part II, "Good Diet, Bad Absorption," Drs. Stephen B. Inkeles, M.D., and Allan Sosin, M.D., discuss how to prevent and treat diabetes Types I and II.

Dr. Anil Minocha, M.D., a gastroenterologist, shares his personal strategies to stave off heartburn. Rohit Medhekar, Ph.D., provides his knowledge on how digestive enzymes play a role in your digestive tract.

Gastroenterologist Dr. Stephen Holt, M.D., says, "Digestive health is considered to be at the root of all general health in the body. It's responsible for the assimilation of nutrients. Without normal absorption, you may have nutrient deficiencies that affect any system in the body structure." He gives insight into irritable bowel syndrome. Dr. Robyn Karlstadt, M.D., discusses basic treatment for ulcers and constipation, while Dr. Trent W. Nichols provides natural treatments to soothe a savage stomach.

6

Diabetes

CONTROLLING DIABETES WITH DR. INKELES'S PLAN

STEPHEN B. INKELES, M.D.

Dr. Stephen Inkeles, who was the director of clinical nutrition at the former Pritikin Longevity Center, has a good handle on how the right diet and supplements can help to prevent and treat diabetes. This all-too-common disease is characterized by elevated levels of blood sugar, or glucose, which results from the body's inability to make enough insulin, a hormone needed to convert sugar, starches, and other food into energy.

So why does Dr. Inkeles have an interest in diabetes? "Number one, I have personal family history of the disease [which can raise your risk of developing diabetes]. Number two, I was impressed with the therapeutic power of lifestyle intervention," says Dr. Inkeles, who told me that his own father developed Type II diabetes at 50 and it was a major contributing cause to his death.

The telltale signs of diabetes may include hunger, unusual thirst, blurred vision, frequent urination, weight loss, and fatigue. If you have any of these symptoms, consult with your doctor.

FACTS F.Y.I.

According to the American Diabetes Association:

- An estimated 17 million Americans have diabetes.
- Type I diabetes usually affects young people and requires insulin treatment. An estimated one million, or 5 to 10 percent of, Americans have Type I.
- Type II diabetes usually develops after age 40. An estimated 16 million, or 90 to 95 percent of, Americans have Type II.

TYPE I AND TYPE II DIABETES

While insulin therapy is needed for Type I diabetes, at Pritikin, patients used more sophisticated types of insulin regimens with meticulous self-monitoring of blood sugars to help them adjust their insulin, explains Dr. Inkeles. Insulin requirements still will go down in Type I with a good diet and exercise program, but it will always be partial; it will never be 100 percent with some of the Type II's that get on insulin. Translation: Type I diabetics have to inject insulin every day because they have zero insulin production themselves.

The good news, however, is that most people who have Type II diabetes can usually control the disease by diet and lifestyle changes.

HOW DIET CAN LOWER YOUR RISK

- *Eat more fiber-rich foods.* Dietary fiber has been associated with reduced insulin requirement in many studies over the past several decades. It is linked with blood sugar control.
- *Lower dietary fat.* A high-fat diet seems to increase the risk of diabetes. Eating five or six mini low-fat, high-fiber meals

will help you to maintain satiety throughout the day to avoid hunger pangs. "Frequent meal eating has been associated with reduction in the development of diabetes, and in somebody with diabetes it's a critical part of their long-term weight loss program," says Dr. Inkeles. And it's believed that the higher your weight, the higher your risk of diabetes.

• *Get a move on.* Regular exercise can help you keep your weight in check. Aerobics and resistance exercise (two to three times per week) can help you change the proportion of muscle to fat, which makes you a better calorie-burning machine, says Dr. Inkeles. The ideal prescription is 45 to 60 minutes of moderate aerobic exercise: an hour of a brisk walk every day seven days a week. "Another way to think of the physiological effect of exercise in diabetic control of blood sugar and making your insulin work better is that exercise lasts about 24 hours."

FOLLOWING A PREVENTIVE APPROACH

Since Dr. Inkeles's dad developed Type II diabetes, the preventive health care doctor himself practices what he preaches to his diabetic patients. His approach includes a "fishatarian" diet, which is plant-based, low-fat, full of whole grains, legumes, fruits, and vegetables, but with an almost complete absence of full-fat dairy products, red meat, and poultry, but liberal amounts of fish.

"It's the exercise component that I've been struggling with in recent months in terms of my weekly frequency. I am, however, quite hopeful that with my forthcoming job change [he is starting his own medical practice], I will have the time to reinstitute my daily walking with brief bouts of running," he told me.

"I do in fact take a variety of supplements, including all those I note as nutraceutically supportive for people with diabetes. However, the dosage strengths I use are more conservative as I'm using them more as part of an overall preventive approach," concludes Dr. Inkeles.

THE DOC'S SUPPLEMENT LIST

Dr. Inkeles recommends these supplements to people who have either Type I or II diabetes.

Supplement	What It Does
Vitamin C	The antioxidant vitamin C helps restore the tissue deficiencies commonly seen in diabetes and helps to inhibit some of the long-term complications of the disease
Magnesium	A mineral that aids in blood sugar control; in the long term it helps reduce the development of diabetic damage to the retina of the eye
Chromium	A mineral that reduces your insulin requirement so that you won't need as much insulin to control your sugar
Alpha-lipoic acid	An antioxidant that improves blood sugar control and can prevent or alleviate the painful diabetic damage to the peripheral nerves

Safety Smarts: Vitamin C: If you take too much, it can cause gastrointestinal problems. Alpha-lipoic acid: If you are diabetic and taking insulin, lipoic acid can lower your blood glucose level, which may lower your need for medications. Talk to your doctor.

DR. SOSIN'S STRATEGIES FOR KIDS

ALLAN SOSIN, M.D.

When I spoke with Allan Sosin, M.D., author of *The Doctor's Guide to Diabetes and Your Child: New Therapies for Type I and*

Type II (Kensington), I was quickly smitten by his earthy style. He reminded me of the unforgettable doctor who made a house call to troubleshoot a boy suffering from asthma in the film *As Good As It Gets*. The fact is, Dr. Sosin comes off real and has a natural flair for caring about people.

As an internist, while Dr. Sosin treats people with all types of diseases, he does treat some children with diabetes. His interest stems from the fact that "they're not treated correctly. And that was just a very powerful impression I got from seeing children with diabetes. They weren't given the right kind of diet, or put on nutritional supplements. The parents didn't understand what the best thing to do was for their kids and they were all very nervous and upset about the situation. It was just out of hand," he explains. Dr. Sosin says he believes while kids with Type I diabetes need insulin, nutritional supplementation plays an important role, too.

MAKING LIFESTYLE CHANGES

"Exercise is important. It works independently of insulin to control the blood sugar. It helps maintain appropriate body weight. One-third of the kids today are overweight, and being overweight contributes to developing diabetes," explains Dr. Sosin.

He adds, "There's a difference between children's diabetes and adult diabetes. Most kids get insulin-deficient diabetes (meaning the pancreas is damaged). But what happens as people get older is that they develop this Type II diabetes, which relates to insulin resistance. And a lot of what my book is about as well is putting kids into the right kind of lifestyle to prevent them from developing diabetes when they become adults." And this is important since the incidence of diabetes is going up all the time.

Keep in mind, "There is a strong genetic predisposition if you have a first-degree relative (mother, father, sister, or brother) with diabetes. Your chance of getting it is about 50 percent," says Dr. Sosin.

However, this is modifiable by lifestyle. "The reason that so many new people are getting it is not because the genetics have changed, but because the lifestyle has changed. As the population gets heavier they get more insulin resistant and the blood sugar goes up and in order to prevent or treat it, you work on exercise, having people on a low–glycemic index diet," explains Dr. Sosin.

He says the glycemic index relates to refined carbohydrates— the foods that tend to cause the most elevation of blood sugar when you eat them and cause the body to require insulin. So you want to avoid high-glycemic foods such as white bread, pasta, potatoes, fruit juices, soft drinks, and fast foods.

And most importantly, diabetes can be eliminated. "It's a reversible problem. It can be cured," says Dr. Sosin, whose mother-in-law and sister-in-law are affected by diabetes. "My sister-in-law's blood sugar has been brought down to normal; and my mother-in-law's blood sugar is approaching normal," says Dr. Sosin. The reason: They have been following what the doctor recommends for treatment and prevention of diabetes.

The catch is, "It's a lot of work changing your life around," points out Dr. Sosin. "So folks who are used to going to Burger King and McDonald's four or five times a week, or drinking five or six Cokes a week, have to make some changes. And people who are not exercising need to do that on a daily basis." He concludes, "Diabetes is not only sweeping the nation, it's sweeping the world. There's going to be 250 million people with diabetes in ten years."

THE DOC'S SUPPLEMENT LIST

Here are some supplements Dr. Sosin recommends to prevent and treat diabetes I and II.

Supplement	What It Does
Alpha-lipoic acid	Antioxidant to control the blood sugar; helps prevent oxidative damage due to the elevated blood sugar so it can help protect the eys and nerves

Magnesium	An important mineral for heart function that can help fight the hardening of the arteries caused by diabetes
CoQ_{10}	Fat-soluble compound that acts like an antioxidant, enhancing the reaction of insulin; it reduces the oxidative damage that the diabetes causes
Essential fatty acids (omega-3s)	It helps control the blood sugar and helps prevent damage to all tissues

Safety Smarts: Alpha-lipoic acid: If you are diabetic and taking insulin, lipoic acid can lower your blood glucose level, which may lower your need for medications. Talk to your doctor. Omega-3 oils: Don't take high doses of fish oil capsules if you are taking NSAIDs (nonsteroidal anti-inflammatory drugs). It may increase gastrointestinal ulcers or bleeding.

DR. TILLOTSON'S SMART SOLUTIONS

ALAN TILLOTSON, PH.D.

One night when I was writing a health article on headaches, I interviewed Dr. Alan Tillotson for his expertise on herbal remedies. During our conversation, the doctor, an herbal wizard, told me that he was diagnosed with Type I diabetes in 1961 at the age of 11.

"Now, almost 40 years later, I have not suffered any major diabetes-related health problems," he told me. By turning to natural therapies, including herbs, Dr. Tillotson has managed to stop all problems associated with diabetes.

THE DOC'S SUPPLEMENT LIST

Here's a selection of herbs that Dr. Tillotson uses himself or recommends to diabetics. You can get a complete list of tips for diabetics in his book *The One Earth Herbal Sourcebook* (Kensington).

Supplement	What It Does
Bilberry extract (blueberries)	This nutrient staves off vascular, or blood vessel, damage in diabetics; it contains anthocyanins, plant chemicals that help repair tiny blood vessels especially in the eyes
Garlic	This herb can help promote digestion
Siberian ginseng root bark	This herb can regulate and lower elevated blood sugars

Safety Smarts: Garlic: Do not use garlic before or after surgery (it's a blood thinner). If you are already taking blood-thinning medications or aspirin, consult with your doctor first.

DOC'S RX TO HEAL YOURSELF

- Take alpha-lipoic acid and essential fatty acids to control blood sugar.
- Use CoQ_{10} to enhance the reaction of insulin.
- Exercise to help control blood sugar.
- Forgo fast food and refined sugar, opting for a healthful, nutrient-dense diet.
- Try herbal remedies such as Siberian ginseng and garlic to help prevent diabetic complications.

Bios

Stephen B. Inkeles, M.D., M.P.H., received his medical degree from the Loyola University of Chicago in Maywood, Illinois. He is a diplomate of both the American Board of Internal Medicine and the American Board of Nutrition. He was a full-time staff physician and director of clinical nutrition at the former Pritikin Longevity Center in Santa Monica, California; and he currently has his own medical practice in Beverly Hills, California. He is 48, is married, has two children, and lives in Malibu, California.

Allan Sosin, M.D., is an internal medicine specialist who is the director of the Institute of Progressive Medicine. As a graduate of Northwestern University, he is one of the leading alternative medical authorities on diabetes in children and teens. He works and lives in Irvine, California. At 56, he is married and has three children.

Alan Tillotson, Ph.D., is a medical herbalist. He received his Ph.D. from International University in Maui, Hawaii. He owns his own practice in Wilmington, Delware. At 50, he is married and has one child. Web site: www.OneEarthHerbs.com.

7

Heartburn

FIGHTING HEARTBURN WITH DR. MINOCHA

ANIL MINOCHA, M.D.

Chronic acid reflux or heartburn affects people of all ages. However, in many cases making easy lifestyle changes is all that is needed to get rid of this problem, according to gastroenterologist Dr. Anil Minocha, author of *How to Stop Heartburn* (John Wiley & Sons).

Here is Dr. Minocha's personal six-step plan for keeping heartburn at bay, which can work for you:

1. Eat only when you are calm and not in a rush. Eat small, frequent meals. Avoid large meals, and stop eating when you feel full.
2. Avoid eating or drinking foods that promote reflux. Stay clear of mint, onions, chocolate, tomatoes, beans, and cabbage. Don't drink alcohol, and avoid orange and grapefruit juice, coffee, and carbonated beverages. Mixed drinks like a bloody mary, grasshopper, or sangria are a double whammy for heartburn sufferers and far worse than a simple glass of

white wine. Heartburn sufferers should drink fluids in the form of water, skim or low-fat milk, or apricot juice. If you must have carbonated beverages, drink 7-Up or Sprite.

3. Quit smoking. Smoking increases acid reflux and delays healing of the acid-induced injury of the food pipe.

4. Do not sleep for about two hours after a meal. Raising the head end of the bed about six inches by placing a block underneath uses gravity to decrease or prevent acid reflux as well as clear any refluxed material soon after it goes into the esophagus. (Pillows are not an alternative.)

5. Your weight matters. There is much more pressure on the stomach in overweight people, leading to increased reflux. Eat healthy foods and exercise to optimize your weight.

6. Don't allow yourself to be stressed easily. Relaxation exercises reduce heartburn and reflux.

Remember, effective medical treatments are available for those that cannot be helped by above measures. Talk to your doctor.

FACTS F.Y.I.

According to Dr. Minocha:

- Heartburn affects 60 million Americans.
- As many as 80 percent of pregnant women suffer from it.
- Infants who have heartburn usually outgrow it by the time they are about 18 months old.
- Heartburn is more common among the elderly, and they also tend to have more complications.

RESEARCH IN A NUTSHELL

According to a survey (based on 1,000 Americans and released August 24, 2000) by the American Gastroenterological Association:

- About 75 percent of those people who suffer nighttime heartburn claim the symptoms keep them awake.
- Close to 50 million people experience nighttime heartburn at least one time per week.
- Roughly 45 million people endure nighttime symptoms that "negatively impact" their sleep.

SECOND OPINION: DR. MEDHEKAR'S ENZYME THERAPY

ROHIT MEDHEKAR, PH.D.

You may already know that enzymes in our body help promote good digestion. However, it may be news to you that unless you live on an all-raw diet, digestive enzyme supplements could enhance both your digestion and good health.

Rohit Medhekar, Ph.D., a researcher, knows firsthand how to keep enzymatically healthy. He told me exactly how enzymes help speed up digestion and help you to absorb essential vitamins and minerals from the food you eat. Not only does this doctor know about the role enzymes play in digestion, he personally takes a digestive enzyme with his meals to ensure good digestion.

Simply put, digestive enzymes provide digestive support. An enzyme is a biochemical catalyst. Like little Pacmen, enzymes can speed up the digestive process and break down the food so your body can absorb it, explains Dr. Medhekar.

In addition, digestive enzymes may help to prevent heartburn. "If your small intestine is not digesting the food, the food will stay in the stomach longer. As long as there is food in the stomach, acid will be produced. When that acid gets into the esophagus it can cause heartburn. So the faster the food gets out of your stomach, the better."

Why? Why does such a young, healthy doctor take digestive enzymes? "I eat only cooked food," he answers. "Well, I eat a salad once in a while," he says adding, "I refuse to eat meat raw." And the fact is, many of us opt for the typical Western diet, which is cooked and processed. Any food that is not raw is enzyme-depleted, which can contribute to poor digestion and disease.

He turns to digestive enzymes to maintain the function of his pancreas. "I don't want to overtax my pancreas. I don't want to overwork my digestive system. Any time you overwork anything it's going to break down," he says adding that he takes a multiple enyzme supplement as a digestive preventive aid. (For more information about enzymes, log onto www.enzymeuniversity.com.)

THE DOC'S SUPPLEMENT LIST

Dr. Medhekar takes digestive enzymes and recommends them to anyone who doesn't live on sprouts.

Supplement	What It Does
Digestive enzymes	Helps you to digest your food faster and more efficiently; plus, it can get rid of stomach acid, a cause of heartburn

DOCS' RX TO HEAL YOURSELF

- Eat your meals s-lo-w-l-y.
- Stay clear of heartburn trigger foods.
- Nix nicotine.
- Don't get your z's after eating a meal.
- Chill out.
- Opt for digestive enzyme supplements to ensure good digestion.

BIOS

Rohit Medhekar, Ph.D., is a researcher at National Enzyme Company in Forsyth, Missouri. A graduate of the University of

Iowa, at 30, he is single and currently resides in Springfield, Missouri.

Anil Minocha, M.D., is board certified in gastroenterology, internal medicine and geriatrics. He is chief of gastroenterology at Southern Illinois University School of Medicine. He attended Government Medical College in Rohtak, India. He also received additional schooling and training at Baylor College of Medicine in Houston and other colleges. Dr. Minocha is the author of *2000 Minocha's Guide to Digestive Diseases* (International Medical Publishing). At 44, he resides in Illinois. Web site: www.diagnosis health.com. and www.geocities.com/aminocha.

8

Irritable Bowel Syndrome

STEPHEN HOLT, M.D.

Irritable bowel syndrome (IBS) is a common gastrointestinal disorder. Symptoms can include abdominal pain or cramping and changes in bowel function such as bloating, gas, diarrhea, and constipation.

In fact, during graduate school I had frequent bouts of IBS, which I blame partially on the stress of scheduling back-to-back classes. Interestingly, Dr. Stephen Holt, M.D., unlike some conventional doctors, is well aware of the mind-body link and how it can bring on a bout of IBS. Too bad he wasn't my doctor back then, because his suggestions could have been helpful.

"It's important that IBS sufferers understand what this disease is, what factors can cause it, and why the manifestation occurs in the first place. The things that I believe that are very valuble are natural approaches":

- *Fiber isn't enough.* "Supplementation of dietary fiber in IBS is quite useful at relieving symptoms of incomplete evacuation of the bowels," points out Dr. Holt, "but it is often in-effective for the control of abdominal pain."

When Dr. Holt told me this it brought back memories of when I was in graduate school. I made an appointment with a gastroenterologist. I explained to the doctor that having too many classes and not enough time was affecting my reg-ularity. As he wrote down several high-fiber foods for me to eat I said, "But what about my stomach? It hurts." He just ignored me. Nor did he address my incredible stress load. However, Dr. Holt understands the mind-body link in IBS patients.

- *Smooth muscle relaxer (natural or synthetic origin).* This will help your smooth muscle (the muscle in your intestinal wall) immediately with the symptoms such as spasm in the bowel. "You can use things like peppermint oil or go to drugs and try antispasmodic drugs."

- *Destress yourself.* Stress can cause grumbling guts, accord-ing to Dr. Holt, author of *Natural Ways to Digestive Health* (M. Evans). The mind-body connection has been linked to gastrointestinal disorders such as IBS.

He adds that many destressing techniques can affect the gut-mind, including hypnotherapy, music therapy, prayer, chiropractic, tough therapy, exercise, and yoga. All of these can help to relax the mind and stomach.

RESEARCH IN A NUTSHELL

When your stomach is upset, that's when you can turn to friendly bacteria supplements called probiotics—the opposite of antibiotics (the most common include acidophilus and bifidobac-teria)—which can help relieve symptoms from the lack of good bacteria. Researchers know that there are multiple benefits of friendly bacteria such as helping absorption of food and miner-als, improving the gut immune system, and getting rid of diges-tion disorders: colitis, peptic ulcer, and IBS.

In a four-week double-blind placebo-controlled trial of 60 people with IBS, treatment with probiotics lessened intestinal gas significantly. The results persisted for one year after treatment was stopped. (Nobaek S, Johansson M-L, Molin G, et al. "Alteration of intestinal microflora is associated with reduction in abdominal bloating and pain in patients with irritable bowel syndrome." *American Journal of Gastroenterology.* 2000; 95:1231–1238)

THE DOC'S SUPPLEMENT LIST

Dr. Holt recommends these supplements to people who suffer from IBS symptoms.

Supplement	What It Does
Fiber	Fiber supplements can relieve symptoms of incomplete evacuation of the bowels
Peppermint oil	Can relax spasm in the bowel
Probiotics	Get rid of IBS symptoms such as intestinal gas

Safety Smarts: Peppermint can cause heartburn.

DOC'S RX TO HEAL YOURSELF

- Include an adequate amount of dietary fiber in your daily diet, at least 25 to 35 grams per day.
- You may want to try peppermint oil to relax spasm in the bowel.
- Probiotics can help get rid of digestive disorders such as IBS.
- Try destressing techniques such as yoga and meditation to relax the mind and the stomach.

BIO

Stephen Holt, M.D., is a leading expert in the field of health and preventive medicine. He graduated from the University of Liverpool Medical School in England. Board certified in internal medicine and gastroeneterology, Dr. Holt practices medicine in New York. He is also a researcher and teacher as well as the author of several books including *The Soy Revolution* (Dell). He lives in New York, is 50-something, is married, and has five children.

9

Gastrointestinal Problems

DR. NICHOLS'S NATURAL PRESCRIPTION

TRENT W. NICHOLS, M.D.

Dr. Trent W. Nichols, a savvy gastroenterologist and author of *Optimal Digestion* (HarperCollins), knows his stomach stuff. In fact, recently I was assigned an article on digestion and I turned to him A.S.A.P. and got immediate results.

I've been considering going south of the border to Mexico but have a major fear of getting sick. After all, an estimated 60 to 70 million Americans suffer from stomach problems, according to the National Institute of Diabetes and Digestive and Kidney Diseases in Bethesda, Maryland. What if I experienced stomach pain, bloating, gas, or diarrhea—common symptoms of digestive disorders sometimes caused by the water or food in Mexico? But Dr. Nichols set me straight. He told me to take bismuth-containing preparations (Pepto Bismol–type products) and to have a good time.

THE DOC'S SUPPLEMENT LIST

Here, take a look at 12 natural supplemental strategies that Dr. Nichols uses for himself, his family, and his patients to prevent and treat a variety of common digestive woes.

Disorder	Supplement	What It Does
Celiac disease (an extreme allergy to protein found in wheat)	Glutamine, an amino acid (supplement)	Helps to heal the small intestine and reduces leaky gut (improper function of the small intestine)
Constipation	Magnesium (supplement)	Smooth muscle relaxer; speeds up the passage of food throughout the entire intestinal tract
Diarrhea	Probiotics (supplement)	Restores good bacteria and destroys the bad bacteria that often causes diarrhea and yeast infections
Diverticulitis (inflammation of pockets that occur inside the wall of the colon where it's stretched out)	Spearmint or peppermint (tea or capsules)	It relaxes the smooth muscle so it doesn't get tense or tight
Gallstones (bile concentrates that form a stone)	Bear bile (the bile from bears; a Chinese extract)	It helps dissolve the stone; alleviates gallbladder disease

Heartburn	Mastic gum (an herbal remedy)	It aids in getting rid of bacteria that cause inflammation of the stomach
Hemorrhoids	Aloe vera (oral; suppository)	Anti-inflammatory
Inflammatory bowel disease	Omega-3 fatty acid (supplement)	Restores vitamin A for antibody production
Irritable bowel syndrome	Peppermint (tea or capsule)	Antispasmodic that relieves a spastic colon
Lactose intolerance	An enzyme replacement	Replaces you're missing lactase, which breaks down the milk sugar so you don't get bloating, gas, or diarrhea
Leaky gut syndrome	Bioactive peptide (made from deepsea white fish such as hake or pollack)	It helps the small intestine grow and aids in inflammation; helps restore the cell lining of your gut
Ulcers	Bismuth-containing preparations	Gets rid of the bad bacteria; heals the gut lining

Safety Smarts: Peppermint: Too much can cause heartburn. Omega fish oils: Don't take high doses of fish oil capsules if you are taking NSAIDs (nonsteroidal anti-inflammatory drugs). It may increase gastrointestinal ulcers and bleeding.

DOCTOR'S LINGO

Good Bacteria: When we don't eat right, take antibiotics, are exposed to environmental toxins, or abuse alcohol, we can destroy the good bacteria in our body, allowing bad bacteria to invade. The best way to restock the body with good bacteria is to eat fermented dairy products, especially yogurt with live and active cultures that contain good bacteria called probiotics (which means "for life"). Probiotics aid digestion, produce important nutrients, and get rid of toxins in the body. Yogurt is easily digested and absorbed. Or turn to probiotic supplements such as *Lactobacillus acidophilus*, which produce an antibacterial substance that can kill several kinds of bacteria, including *E. coli*, *Streptococcus*, and *Salmonella*, according to medical experts. Probiotic supplements can help relieve the symptoms caused by the lack of good bacteria.

SECOND OPINION: DR. KARLSTADT'S PRACTICAL REMEDIES

ROBYN KARLSTADT, M.D.

It doesn't take a rocket scientist to figure out that gastroenterologist Dr. Robyn Karlstadt takes the conservative approach when it comes to stomach woes. Here's the doctor's lowdown on ulcers and constipation—two problems that people don't like to discuss or have to cope with!

Ulcers? No Problem!

"Currently, stomach ulcers appear to be related most commonly to a bacterial infection. Therefore, if someone has abdominal pain and is diagnosed (with X-ray or endoscopy) with an ulcer, the patient may be placed on a one- to two-week antibiotic regimen," she explains.

Adds Dr. Karlstadt: "The other 10 percent of ulcers are most frequently associated with the use of aspirin or nonsteroidal anti-inflammatory agents, which can be purchased over the counter. Therefore, if a person is experiencing discomfort when taking these medications, he should stop them. Occasional use is usually not a problem, but continual daily use may lead to excess irritation in the stomach, leading to ulceration or bleeding." Best advice: Whenever you use an anti-inflammatory drug, do what Dr. Karlstadt does: Make sure that you eat or have just eaten. Food serves as a buffer.

Say Goodbye to Constipation

Irregularity may be caused by a number of things, says Dr. Karlstadt. "Women have slower gut transit times than men and may be slightly more prone to constipation," she points out.

"When I was younger, I ate more junk food, and was not as active. I did have constipation as a problem. At that time, I would eat prunes, which definitely did help—but I feel much healthier now!" Here are the doctor's personal tips:

- *Drink six to eight glasses of water a day.* Water helps to keep your system regular.
- *Eat two to three servings of fruits and two to three servings of vegetables daily.* These also help keep your system regular. What's more, the American Cancer Society notes that eating fruits and vegetables may help reduce the risk of developing colon cancer.
- *Do moderate exercise daily.* Exercise also keeps the system regular. "I lift weights and do cross-training three alternate days a week. I jump rope (about a thousand jumps) or do aerobic walking on alternate days."

RESEARCH IN A NUTSHELL

The old school of thought, explains Dr. Karlstadt, was that ulcers were caused by too much stomach acid. Today, researchers blame a bacterium called *Helicobacter pylori*. This bacterium has been identified in 79 to 90 percent of ulcer sufferers. When it's present, the mucous layer of the stomach is digested and acid comes into close contact with the unprotected lining. That's why the latest approach is to kill *H. pylori* with antibiotics. (Ken Babal, *Good Digestion*, Alive Books, 2000, p. 32)

DOCS' RX TO HEAL YOURSELF

- Consider natural digestive aids such as vitamins and supplements to prevent and treat digestive problems.
- Opt for herbs such as peppermint and spearmint to soothe heartburn and relax the smooth muscle.
- Use digestive enzyme supplements for lactose intolerance and to ensure good digestion.
- Turn to probiotics when you have diarrhea or need to restock your body with good bacteria.
- If you must take an anti-inflammatory drug, make sure that you eat food to buffer your stomach.
- To stay regular, eat a fiber-rich diet, drink plenty of water, and get regular exercise.

BIOS

Robyn Karlstadt, M.D., is an internist and gastroenterologist. She is senior director of global medical affairs at Wyeth-Ayerst Laboratories in St. Davids, Pennsylvania. She attended Boston University School of Medicine. She resides in southern New Jersey, is married, and has two children.

Trent W. Nichols, M.D., is a gastroenterologist who has a practice in Hanover, Pennsylvania. He graduated from Northwestern University in Chicago, Illinois. At 57, he is married, has one child and lives in Hanover, Pennsylvania. Web site: gutdoc.org.

PART III

From Colds to Cancer

A few years ago, I had a bad case of flu. My doctor prescribed bed rest—and a nurturing caretaker. I went home, plopped on the couch, pulled up the comforter, and waited for my dear surrogate grandmother to pay me a visit. She is an elderly woman who always has been there for me in the best and worst of times.

Ginny helped comfort me. And her home remedies, vitamin C and herbal teas, worked like a strong antibiotic that night and throughout the weekend. The natural wonders she gave me helped me get back on the road to a speedy recovery.

This comes as no news to the doctors in Part III, "From Colds to Cancer," who say diet, supplements, and lifestyle can help bolster the immune system.

Drs. Kenneth Bock and Andrew Weinstein recommend natural prevention and treatment of both allergies and asthma—both linked to your immune system.

Speaking of the immune system . . . In the cancer section some of the doctors I interviewed include James A. Duke, Ph.D., who shines herbal light on cancer from a personal perspective, while oncologist James W. Forsythe, M.D., shares his cancer-fighting nutrients, and cancer survivor Jack Stephens, D.V.M., provides his foolproof prescription.

Colds and flu are discussed by Dr. Ray Sahelian, author of *The*

Common Cold Cure (Avery). If you've ever wondered what to do when your child has a fever, Dr. Marc Childs dispels myths and provides facts to settle your concerns.

To fight fatigue, listen to Dr. Edward Conley. And if you, or someone you know, is battling aches and pains, Dr. Richard Podell can help with an anti-fibromyalgia plan. Dr. Michael E. Rosenbaum wraps up Part III and discusses the importance of immunity.

10

Allergies and Asthma

DR. BOCK'S ALLERGY ATTACK

KENNETH BOCK, M.D.

Allergy sufferers look forward to spring's allergies about as much as they do to getting a root canal. At this time of year, airborne tree and grass pollen make their lives miserable.

Welcome to the cruel world of allergies, which torment millions of Americans. An estimated 50 percent of Dr. Kenneth Bock's patients are allergy sufferers. Dr. Bock sees all types of allergy and asthma sufferers, so he has a strong expertise in allergies.

FACTS F.Y.I.

According to the American Academy of Allergy, Asthma and Immunology:

- An estimated 38 percent of Americans have at least one allergy.

- Seasonal allergic rhinitis, the wheezing, sneezing, inhalant allergies more commonly called hayfever, affect 35.9 million Americans.
- It is estimated that 12 million Americans suffer from food allergies.
- Allergies can increase the risk of asthma, which afflicts more than 17 million Americans.

COMMON ALLERGIES AND PREVENTION

Inhalant Allergies. Air pollution, dust mites, and animal dander can all trigger allergies or other respiratory ailments in any season. "With allergies you're looking at things that can modulate the immune system, not only build it up. Any type of allergy or hypersensitivity comes from overreactivity of the immune system. So you're looking to quiet it down," explains Dr. Bock.

Rx. There are things you can do other than be anti-cat, avoid cities, and try to eliminate the microscopic critters that infest your home. Antioxidants including vitamins C and E may help quench free radicals that may contribute to inflamed airways. Quercetin can act as a natural antihistamine and inhibit histamine release from mast cells (cells that produce histamines).

Chemical Sensitivities. According to Dr. Bock, people have more chemical sensitivities today than ever before. "There are more chemicals in the environment," he says. "Also our immune systems are exposed to the chemicals, and it is very well known that there is a huge increase in asthma." Chemical sensitivity is difficult to diagnose but, in his opinion, a real problem. (A doctor can test you for immune responses to certain chemicals.)

Rx. Avoid culprits such as aerosol sprays, tobacco smoke, glues, insecticides and herbicides, household chemicals, and fragrances. Identification and avoidance are key, according to Dr. Bock. Vitamin C can help to detoxify adverse chemical reactions in your body.

Food Allergies. The most common food allergens include fish and shellfish, legumes, peanuts, eggs, chocolate, cow's milk, citrus fruits, tomatoes, soy, and wheat. Dr. Bock, for instance, noticed that after large meals of wheat-laden pasta he suffered from fatigue and bloating. To remedy this problem the doctor began to eat more protein, fewer carbs, and saw some improvement.

Rx. If you can't pinpoint which food makes you sick, there are three types of allergy tests that can help you: the skin test, which shows the degree of inflammation after the skin is pricked and exposed to an extract of the suspect food; the elimination diet, to find out whether allergic symptoms disappear when a particular food is removed from your diet; the RAST or ELISA blood test, which evaluates levels of allergy antibodies after a patient's blood is incubated with a suspected food.

THE DOC'S SUPPLEMENT LIST

Dr. Bock takes these supplements to maintain proper immune system balance and to stave off potential allergies and sensitivities.

Supplement	What It Does
Vitamin C	An antioxidant vitamin that can help to detoxify chemicals, which makes it a good defense against allergies; it can help to balance your immune system responses
Vitamin E	An antioxidant vitamin that helps quench free radicals that contribute to inflamed airways
Quercetin	An anti-allergic flavonoid which inhibits hista-

mine release from mast cells and slows the production of other allergy-related compounds; it stabilizes mast cell membranes

Magnesium A mineral that relaxes bronchial tissues, which can help aid allergies and asthma

Omega-3 fatty acids Essential fatty acids can serve as precursors for anti-inflammatory substances in the body such as prostaglandins (remember, inflammation is one of the problems that contribute to asthma)

Safety Smarts: If you take too much vitamin C, it can cause gastrointestinal problems. Omega-3 oils: Don't take high doses of fish oil capsules if you are taking NSAIDs (nonsteroidal anti-inflammatory drugs). It may increase gastrointestinal ulcers and bleeding.

SECOND OPINION: DR. ROYAL'S HOMEOPATHIC REMEDIES

DAN ROYAL, D.O.

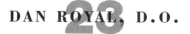

These days, Dr. Dan Royal treats allergies as part of his practice. He provides tests for allergies—food, chemical and pesticides, and inhalant—something he has encountered in the past in his own life. More interesting, he turns to homeopathy (an alternative therapy that works on the premise "like cures like") for himself and his patients.

Dr. Royal told me about his own allergic response, which he experienced years ago at age 17 back in the 1970s, when he lived in Oregon.

"It was a hay fever allergy to grass pollen. It is very common. I noticed it when I mowed the lawn, usually in the summertime. My eyes would get itchy, swollen, and red and I would sneeze. Those are all symptoms common to hay fever," he explains.

Rather than turn to an over-the-counter antihistamine, Dr. Royal took the natural route and turned to his father, a doctor who used homeopathic medicine to treat people with allergies. "They used electrodermal testing (a skin resistance test that is performed on the acupuncture control measurement points and is a type of a biofeedback between operator and patient) to find a combination homeopathic for grass and tree pollen. I started taking homeopathic injections two or three times a week," he recalls, adding that the homeopathic anti-allergy remedy helped to keep his allergy under control.

Three years later, when Dr. Royal had moved to Nevada, he says, "I had the allergies even worse than I had in Oregon. I did the same thing. I went to a clinic where they were able to diagnose me through electrodermal testing and make a homeopathic allergy preparation, which I administered myself by injection. And I did that every day for two weeks. By the end of two weeks my allergies were gone and I didn't have a problem again for maybe 15 years."

How is a homeopathic treatment better than a drug? "If I had taken an antihistamine, it would have helped because the basic response to allergies is the same. It doesn't matter whether you're reacting to grass pollen or a food, it's the body's release of histamine that gives your body the trouble. What we try to do with homeopathic medicine is to stimulate the body to bring about its own healing—to help the body to deal with the problem a little more effectively."

Adds Dr. Royal, "When you make a homeopathic remedy you're using something that has been diluted and shaken to treat what in pharmacological doses would cause symptoms but you're making a homeopathic to neutralize those symptoms. That's the whole premise behind homeopathy. You use things that are similar to what's causing the symptoms or the exact thing if you can find it, make it homeopathic, and it will have a neutralizing effect. So when you take a homeopathic it's like using Mother Nature's antidote."

Allergy Relief

For the most helpful allergy relief, find out which allergies are wreaking havoc in your body and steer clear of them. Allergy experts recommend:

- *Get rid of dust mites.* Sweep out clutter and have your house power-vacuumed, if necessary. Wash bedding and linens in very hot water.
- *Depollinate your environment.* Flip on the air conditioner to sift out pollen (keep its filter and any forced air registers clean). Exercise indoors. Machine-dry, rather than line-dry, your clothes.
- *Buy a home filter.* This is especially important if you experience dust, pollen, or pet dander allergies.
- *Avoid allergy triggers such as mold and tobacco smoke.*

Dr. Weinstein's Asthma Alleviation

ANDREW WEINSTEIN, M.D.

Allergies can increase the risk of asthma, which afflicts more than 17 million Americans according to the American Academy of Allergy, Asthma and Immunology's latest report. Most people with asthma also suffer allergies, according to Dr. Andrew Weinstein, who told me that this is certainly true in the patients he sees in his practice.

Simply put, asthma is a condition that happens when the main air passages of your lungs and bronchial tubes become inflamed. When the muscles of the bronchial walls tighten and too much mucus is made, it causes your airways to narrow. The result can range from minor wheezing to severe breathing problems.

"The research that I've been doing for 25 years focuses on helping people to adapt to chronic disease, specifically asthma," concludes Dr. Weinstein.

Remember the film *As Good As It Gets?* Helen Hunt plays a mom struggling to take care of her son, who has asthma. He never gets the proper treatment until the right doctor pays a house call. According to Dr. Weinstein, that scenario is on the money.

How do you know if a child or adult has asthma? "We measure lung function in individuals old enough to measure lung function, then give them an inhaled asthma medicine to see if the lung function is improved. When individuals have improvement in lung function after the bronchial dilator medicine is inhaled, that would help to define the individual who has asthma," he explains. Some people with asthma can be treated with inhaled medicine, and some can be put on nonsteroidal anti-iflammatory tablets.

Dr. Weinstein treats both children and adults afflicted with asthma. "Not too many people use family therapy as a way to treat severe asthma," points out Dr. Weinstein, who does just that. And it's vital that parents understand what can trigger an asthma attack.

"Stress is an issue for certain individuals with severe symptoms. Individuals with severe asthma have very inflamed airways. And deep breathing maneuvers such as hyperventilation, crying, or yelling will aggravate the asthma and make it worse," explains Dr. Weinstein. Hearing that, I recall movies where characters with asthma who are under stress will have an asthma attack.

Interestingly, Dr. Weinstein had asthma as a child. Once you have asthma, do you always have it? "You tend to outgrow it, and some people tend to regrow it," he says. For him, "It's exercise-related and I use an inhaler before exercise."

The fact is, "Exercise can be considered a trigger for asthma. What's equivalent for an infant with exercise is the concept of crying-related asthma. Usually, when an infant cries, nothing happens except that the parent reacts. However, a child with severe asthma may set off an asthma attack by crying," explains Dr. Weinstein. And it could end up as an emergency room visit.

PLAN OF ATTACK

- Make sure that the child receives some asthma medication beforehand. "Some parents lose control and the child has too much power in the family because they can control the family by getting upset," adds Dr. Weinstein. In other words, asthma can be used as a manipulation device.
- "We meet with the families and discuss this and find out how the family is doing. Then we offer treatment so that they will eliminate the psychologically induced asthma," says Dr. Weinstein.

RESEARCH IN A NUTSHELL

According to medical experts, when vitamin C is low in the body, an asthma attack alert is on high. Vitamin C carries the major antioxidant load in the airways and therefore contributes to the health of the lungs. Clinical trials since the 1970s have shown that vitamin C supplementation provides significant improvements in respiratory function and asthma symptoms.

DOCS' RX TO HEAL YOURSELF

- Avoid triggers, from grass to dust mites, that can cause inhalant allergies.
- Take antioxidant vitamins C and E to help quench free radicals that may contribute to inflamed airways.
- Identify chemicals that can cause sensitivity and avoid them. Vitamin C can help detoxify chemical reactions in your body.
- If you can't pinpoint which food makes you sick, get an allergy test.
- To maintain proper immune system balance and to stave off

potential allergies and sensitivities, take supplements such as vitamins C and E, quercetin, magnesium, and omega-3s.

- Consider going to a homeopath if you have stubborn inhalant allergies.
- Opt for psychological treatment to avoid an imminent asthma attack in a child.

BIOS

Kenneth Bock, M.D., is board certified in family practice. He received his M.D. with honor at the University of Rochester School of Medicine. At 47, his practice, Rhinebeck Health Center (with a focus in integrative medicine), is in Rhinebeck and Albany, New York. He lives in Bearsville, New York, with his wife and two children. His is the author of *The Road to Immunity* (Pocket Books) and *Natural Relief for Your Child's Asthma* (HarperCollins). Web site: www.rhinebeckhealth.com.

Dan Royal, D.O., practices in Henderson, Nevada. He received his degree at the College of Osteopathic Medicine of the Pacific in Pomona, California. At 42, he is married, has three children, and lives in Las Vegas.

Andrew Weinstein, M.D., is board certified in allergy and immunology. He received his M.D. at the University of Pennsylvania in Philadelphia. Dr. Weinstein has a practice called Asthma and Allergy Care of Delaware in Newark. At 53, he resides in Wilmington, Delaware, is married, and has two children.

Cancer

Dr. Forsythe's Cancer-Preventing Nutrients

JAMES W. FORSYTHE, M.D.

Chances are you've got at least one person in your life that has had cancer. But with the guidance of nutrition-minded doctors like Dr. James W. Forsythe, you can cut your cancer risk up to 60 percent by diet and lifestyle changes.

This oncologist with a heartwarming dedication to his cancer patients has a lot to say about cancer prevention. While training as an internist he was drawn into the world of medical oncology. For the last 30 years, Dr. Forsythe, author of *Alternative Medicine: Definitive Guide to Cancer* (Burton Goldberg Future Press), has been an oncologist. However, it's been 15 years since he turned to alternative care.

"By living in Reno and treating patients who were being treated by homeopaths and naturopaths and seeing their good results, I became impressed and wanted to train myself and learn more." Later, he became a board-certified homeopathic doctor as well as an internist.

These days when cancer patients turn to Dr. Forsythe, a homeopathic oncologist, he gives them four options: conventional treatment, combined therapy (his favorite option), alternative therapy, and comfort or hospice care for the terminally ill.

Is seeing cancer patients, day after day, a wake-up call to follow an anti-cancer plan for himself? "It gives me a feeling for life and death and the importance of living every day to the fullest and appreciating good health," explains Dr. Forsythe. "It teaches you compassion and respect for life."

We know that going low-fat, eating more fiber, and focusing on antioxidant vitamins may help trap free radical molecules that cause normal, noncancerous cells to become cancerous. So every morning the busy oncologist makes a nutrient-dense smoothie for himself and his wife. It contains cancer-fighting ingredients such as flaxseed oil, a raw egg, fresh berries, banana, soy protein powder, and frozen yogurt.

While Dr. Forsythe follows a cancer prevention nutrient program, he adds that he gives his patients a lot of the nutrients that he takes himself—and more—with chemotherapy treatments.

"That helps ease the effects of chemo and ease the toxicity. It also helps build the immune system as the chemo is breaking it down. It lessens the nausea, the hair loss, and the lowering of the blood count. It makes the patients feel a lot better and more energetic."

FACTS F.Y.I.

According to the American Cancer Society:

- Cancer is the second major cause of death (next to heart disease) in America.
- In the United States, one in every four deaths is from cancer.

THE DOC'S SUPPLEMENT LIST

Here are the cancer prevention nutrients that help Dr. Forsythe guard against cancer—and can help you too.

Supplement	What It Does	Protection For
Vitamin C	An antioxidant that boosts good white blood cell production; it gobbles up free radicals; it stimulates natural killer cell production	Stomach, larynx, lung, esophagus
Vitamin E	An antioxidant, it's good for cancers of all types; it helps prevent free radical damage to cells that can lead to abnormal cell growth	Stomach, lung, esophagus, prostate
Beta carotene	Beta carotene in the body can change into retinoic acid, a substance used to treat cancer. It's very useful in skin cancers, cancer of the colon and esophagus	Stomach, larynx, lung, esophagus
Selenium	Fights cancer by preventing cell mutation and repairs damage to cells, boosting the immune system due to its antioxidant effect	Lung, colon
Saw palmetto	An herb that can help to keep the prostate healthy	Prostate

Safety Smarts: Vitamin C: If you take too much, it can cause gastrointestinal problems. Selenium: It can be toxic in high doses (more than 600 mcg per day). Saw palmetto: Do not use until you see a doctor first. If you have an enlarged prostate it's important to exclude prostate cancer before using saw palmetto.

Q & A WITH DR. DUKE

JAMES A. (JIM) DUKE, PH.D.

Years ago I interviewed Jim Duke, Ph.D., for information on herbs for my weekly diet and nutrition column for *Woman's World*. Recently, I reconnected with the herbal guru. While readers use tips from his latest book, *The Green Pharmacy Antiaging Prescriptions* (Rodale), I chose to grill the herbal guru on cancer-fighting herbs. And, ironically, I hit on a subject that is indeed very close to home.

Q. *Why do you feel herbs are so important today in cancer prevention?*
A. Mostly for the antioxidants they provide, but also for the thousands of biologically active and important compounds they contain. Herbs offer many chemicals our genes have known (and come to need in some cases) for millions of years. Modern diet, agricultural selection, and food processing do not provide these. Herbs do.

Q. *Do you personally use herbs to help lower your risk of developing cancer?*
A. Many herbs and fruits and vegetables since twenty-five years ago, when my father died of colon cancer.

Q. *What's the most important cancer-fighting herb or your personal favorite and why?*
A. There is no particular herb. It's best to get many of them, and many different fruits and veggies. The idea of a single remedy is

the simpleminded approach of the pharmaceutical industry. One
expensive silver bullet. Cancer, like malaria, like salmonella, can
outsmart a single pharmaceutical. You're better off with the
herbal shotgun.

**Q. *Do you feel more people will begin to take herbs as a cancer
preventive method?***
A. Yes.

**Q. *Are more people who have cancer turning to herbal treat-
ment? And if so, why?***
A. Some give up on chemo and turn to herbs. Chemo kills cancer
and sometimes the patient. Herbs build up the immune system,
which may kill the cancer, but won't kill the patient.

**Q. *Why do you personally have an interest in cancer and cancer-
fighting herbs?***
A. My father and two of his brothers died of colon cancer at 65.
My older brother, now 80, and my younger brother, age 68, are
clearly genetically targeted for colon cancer. The older brother,
like my mother when she was alive (died at 98 or 99), eschews
doctors and medicine with the same passion that M.D.'s eschew
prescribing herbs. I had two or three polypectomies [removal of
polyps, which may be precursors to colon cancer] and my
younger brother has had even more. But if some other scythe
doesn't decapitate my life, I may face the same decision my
non–herbally inclined brother faced at the beginning of 2001. He
had a foot of his colon removed. The odds are not amusing. Fun
with numbers: fatalities due to hospitals = 250,000 a year; fatalities due to colon cancer = 56,000 a year; fatalities due to herbs =
fewer than 50 (mostly ma huang abuse).

RESEARCH IN A NUTSHELL

Dr. Duke favors green tea as one of his anti-cancer secrets.
Scientists believe the catechins in green tea help to prevent cancer
by lowering the toxicity of certain carcinogens, which may reduce

their cancer-causing potential; interrupt the binding of cancer-causing substances to the DNA of healthy cells; act as antioxidants, which help protect the body against free radical damage; and inhibit tumors from starting. (Nadine Taylor, *Green Tea: The Natural Secret for a Healthier Life* [Kensington, 1998])

What's more, a 1990 study published in *The Japanese Journal of Cancer Research* found that consumption of green tea lowered the risk of colon cancer. (Kato I, Tominagra S, Matsuura A, et al. "A comparative case-control study of colorectal cancer and adenoma." *The Japanese Journal of Cancer Research.* 1990; 81:1101–1108)

THE DOC'S SUPPLEMENT LIST

Dr. Duke eats plenty of anti-cancer nutrient-dense vegetables. Here are some of his favorites in a homemade vegetarian soup:

Nutrient	What It Does	Protection For	Vegetable Source
Beta carotene	In the body, this vitamin can change into retinoic acid, a substance used to treat cancer of the blood and bladder	Stomach, larynx, lung, esophagus, breast	Carrots
Indole-3-carbinols	These chemicals help decrease the "bad" estrogen that causes cancerous mutation in cells	Lungs, colon, breast, bladder	Kale
Quercetin	Functions as an antioxidant	Stomach	Onion

Lycopene	This nutrient helps destroy free radicals	Stomach, colon, mouth throat	Tomato

SECOND OPINION Q & A WITH DR. COWAN

THOMAS COWAN, M.D.

Plenty of people these days may link Iscador with actor and breast cancer survivor Suzanne Somers. That's when I first heard about the controversial herbal treatment for cancer she used.

I called Dr. Thomas Cowan, who sees patients who are battling all different types of cancers. And this general practitioner does indeed offer Iscador, which he knows is controversial but is in demand. He prescribes it to people who suffer from a variety of cancers, from colon to liver cancer, at all ages but very rarely children. Iscador, he says, has no side effects.

Q. What is Iscador?
A. There isn't a category to put it in. It's a very particular pharmaceutical preparation of fermented whole mistletoe plant [which has been used as a medicinal herb for centuries in Europe].

Q. Mistletoe? Holiday mistletoe? How does it work?
A. Yes. You have to have a doctor's prescription to use it. It has mild cytotoxic effects, meaning that it kills cancer cells. And it has a broad-ranging immune stimulation effect. In particular, it increases the number of white blood cells, it increases the temperature, and it increases the amount and activity of natural killer cells.

Q. Can you take it in conjunction with chemotherapy or radiation?
A. Yes. I recommend it to every cancer patient I see. I suggest that

they do mistletoe for a while, at least a year. And whether they should do other things depends on the situation. Less than 10 percent of the time do I tell them they should do only mistletoe.

Q. *Why the ruckus about Suzanne Somers taking Iscador?*
A. It's just pure hysteria. Because in Germany there's at least 300,000 people who are using Iscador therapy.

Q. *Do you see success with Iscador?*
A. I have some people do exceptionally well, and I have some people whom it doesn't seem to help, mostly because their pain [cancer] is too far along. There's only one substance that we know of that is both a cytotoxic agent and an immune stimulant. And that's why mistletoe is so special and unique.

Q. *If you ever got cancer would you use Iscador yourself?*
A. Yes, without a doubt. It's the only natural, non–side effect treatment that is both a cytotoxic and an immune stimulant.

DR. WILLIAMS'S ANTI-CANCER PLAN

DAVID E. WILLIAMS, PH.D.

As a researcher studying the protective effects of phytochemicals and vitamins from fruits and vegetables in the reduction of cancer risk, Dr. David Williams is personally committed to enhancing his daily intake of these important chemicals.

THE DOC'S SUPPLEMENT LIST

Dr. Williams takes these supplements each day to help lower his risk of developing cancer.

Supplement	What It Does	Dosage
Vitamin E	"The vitamins supplement the low anti-oxidant intake I get from not consuming	400 IU

sufficient quantities of fruits and vegetables and provide general protection against cancer influenced by oxidative stress," says Dr. Williams.

Vitamin C		500 mg
Multivitamin		
Selenium	This antioxidant trace mineral provides protection against prostate cancer and perhaps cancers at other sites.	0.2 mg
Baby aspirin	The aspirin is to provide protection against colon cancer.	81 mg

Safety Smarts: Vitamin C: If you take too much, it can cause gastrointestinal problems. Selenium: It can be toxic in high doses (more than 600 mcg per day).

DR. STEPHENS'S PET PRESCRIPTION

JACK STEPHENS, D.V.M.

Back in 1990, Dr. Jack Stephens was diagnosed with oral cancer. During treatments of radiation, chemotherapy, and brachytherapy (in which radiation is implanted around the cancer) the veterinarian realized that Spanky, his wife's miniature pinscher, was having a big impact on his recovery.

"As a cancer survivor, I have experienced the support that a pet unconditionally provides, and how it can affect the mental and physical health of a human," explains Dr. Stephens.

Spanky tuned in to Dr. Stephens' mood swings. On the days when the doctor didn't think he had the energy to get out of bed, Spanky inspired him to get up and go for a walk and heal.

Today, Dr. Stephens is a cancer survivor. While Spanky is no longer around, the doctor has formed another human-canine bond with Skeeter, also a miniature pinscher. Like Spanky, Skeeter is his constant pal. Dr. Stephens is no longer practicing veterinary medicine; however, he is busy at work since he is the founder of Veterinary Pet Insurance.

RESEARCH IN A NUTSHELL

"Through the efforts of the VPI Skeeter Foundation [a nonprofit organization dedicated to demonstrating the positive effects of the human-animal bond], we will help quantify the importance of the human-animal bond," says Dr. Jack Stephens. Heading the Foundation's list for 2001 is the Oldendaal Study.

The Oldendaal Study will find out to what extent chemical changes linked to the human-animal bond occur in older adults and dogs when they become bonded—or not. The study will measure the body's chemicals—such as cortisol (stress hormone), oxytocin (happiness hormone), and endorphin (warm feeling hormone)—before and after the interactions. "We hope the study will prove what we have known for years . . . that the human-animal bond is strong enough to promote positive health and healing," says Dr. Stephens, who has been ill and healed thanks to his canine companion. (Information from the VPI Skeeter Foundation's web site: SkeeterFoundation.org)

DOC'S RX TO HEAL YOURSELF

- Take antioxidant supplements C, E, beta carotene, and selenium to prevent free radical damage to cells that can lead to abnormal cell growth.
- Use the herb saw palmetto to maintain a healthy prostate.
- Eat vegetables that contain cancer-fighting substances such as quercetin, indoles, and lycopene.

- Drink green tea, which may lower the toxicity of cancer-causing substances.
- If you have cancer, consider Iscador, a medicinal herb that can destroy cancer cells and stimulate the immune system.
- The healing power of pets can both prevent and treat cancer by enhancing the immune system.

BIOS

Thomas Cowan, M.D., is a general practitoner in Peterborough, New Hampshire. He went to Michigan State University in East Lansing. At 44, he is married, has three children and one stepchild, and resides in Peterborough.

James A. Duke, Ph.D., is a botanical consultant at Herbal Vineyard, Inc. He is the author of dozens of books on herbs. Dr. Duke is a graduate of the University of North Carolina in Chapel Hill. He lives in Fulton, Maryland, with his wife and has two children. Web site: URL for Father Nature's Farmacy: http://www.ars-grin.gov/duke.

James W. Forsythe, M.D., is board certified in internal medicine, medical oncology, and homeopathy. Dr. Forsythe received his doctorate of medicine at the University of California at San Francisco. He is the founder of the Cancer Screening and Treatment Center of Nevada and a second homeopathic clinic called the Century Wellness Clinic both in Reno, Nevada. At 62, he is married, has five children, and lives in Reno. Web site: www. dr forsythe.com.

Jack Stephens, D.V.M., received his D.V.M. from the University of Missouri College of Veterinary Medicine. Dr. Stephens is founder and chief executive officer of Veterinary Pet Insurance. He is 54 years old, and lives in Anaheim, California, with his wife, children, and stepchildren. Web site: petinsurance.com.

David Williams, Ph.D., is a professor in the department of environmental and molecular toxicology at Oregon State University with an appointment also in the Linus Pauling Institute. He received his Ph.D. from Oregon State University. At 48, he resides in Corvallis, Oregon, with his wife and three children.

12

Colds and Flu

DR. SAHELIAN'S TEN-STEP PREVENTION PLAN

RAY SAHELIAN, M.D.

As a busy journalist always on deadline, I must admit that whenever I need information regarding a health topic, Dr. Ray Sahelian is one of my favorite doctors to turn to. As I see it, his approach as a general practitioner is simple: He personally combines good nutrition with supplements to prevent colds and flu, especially during winter, the height of the cold-and-flu season.

Since he is the author of *The Common Cold Cure* (Avery), he was the perfect doctor to turn to for natural cold and flu remedies. For instance, the last time he noticed a cold starting was two years ago, he says. "I had a little sore throat and some nasal stuffiness. I loaded up on zinc lozenges and stopped it dead in its tracks."

Here are ten natural cold-busters that Dr. Sahelian uses himself and recommends to his patients to keep from getting sick year round.

1. Drink plenty of fluids. Drinking water, herbal teas, and vitamin C–rich liquids can flush out any toxins that you accumulate.

2. Wash your hands frequently. Viruses can be transmitted by shaking someone's hand and then touching your face, nose or mouth, says Dr. Sahelian. He advises you to wash your hands often as a preventive measure.

3. Eat right. All year round Dr. Sahelian tries to eat a good balance of antioxidant-rich fruits and vegetables. "There are many plant chemicals such as carotenoids and flavonoids that have antiviral and antibacterial activity," he says. So eating nutritious produce daily will help you keep your immune system strong 365 days a year. He also eats fish and poultry, legumes, and whole grains, all chock-full of nutrients that keep the immune system strong. Onions and garlic—natural immunity boosters—help stave off colds and flu, too.

4. Treat yourself well. "I try to minimize junk food, but I do succumb to chocolate or calcium-rich ice cream once or twice a week," he says. "It's possible that lots of sugar can interfere with the proper functioning of the immune system."

5. Take vitamin C. "I take half a gram (500 milligrams) a day. Most of the research says that it improves the immune system. Also, at the earliest onset of a cold I recommend taking three to five grams immediately," says Dr. Sahelian, who recommends combining vitamin C with zinc lozenges for extra protection.

6. Take echinacea. This herb, which is touted to have both antibiotic and immune-stimulating properties, is beneficial if you're coming down with a cold. "It may stimulate the immune system to fight off a cold, but the research as far as preventing a cold is not consistent," says Dr. Sahelian.

7. Zinc yourself well. "Zinc lozenges are the most powerful and second is vitamin C," he says. Zinc is a potent virus-fighter that can cut the time you spend in misery. So don't leave home without it—as Dr. Sahelian did. Six years ago Dr. Sahelian had a full-blown cold. He explains, "I was in Alaska way out in the wilderness and I ran out of my zinc after two lozenges. I was in a van traveling with a group of

people. And one of the people sitting in the back had a cold. I couldn't avoid the exposure. All I had left was plenty of tea. I just kept drinking plenty of warm liquid." And it helped.

8. Drink herbal teas. "Warm liquids help loosen mucus," explains Dr. Sahelian.

9. Exercise, exercise, exercise. "I exercise and take long walks almost daily. It helps me to sleep more deeply at night. Deep sleep is a time when the immune system has a chance to regroup itself and get revitalized," explains Dr. Sahelian.

10. Chill out. "I reduce my stress by yoga twice a week," says Dr. Sahelian. He believes that by keeping your stress levels down, you can keep your immune system up and healthy.

Do You Have a Cold or the Flu?

Dr. Sahelian often sees patients complaining of sniffles, coughs, aches, and pains during the height of cold and flu season. These tips—straight from the doctor—can help you to pinpoint the most common respiratory infections if you or your family gets sick.

Illness	Symptoms
Common cold	Runny nose, nasal congestion, sore throat, cough, muscle aches and pains, headache
Strep throat	White mucus on the tonsils or throat, severe sore throat, difficulty swallowing
Acute bronchitis	Cough that causes mucus in the throat and lungs
Influenza	Muscle aches and pains, headaches, low back pain, fatigue, some depression, significant fever

Pneumonia	Fever above 102°F, cough, weakness, thick or bloody phlegm

THE DOC'S SUPPLEMENT LIST

Here are the supplements that Dr. Sahelian turns to when he feels a cold or flu coming on.

Supplement	What It Does
Vitamin C	An antioxidant that supercharges your immune system
Echinacea	An herb that helps white blood cells and T-cells necessary to build up the immune system and stave off infection
Zinc	A mineral that revs up antibody production and helps the body mend damaged membranes that might otherwise let an infection occur; it's best used as a preventive measure, but not on a regular basis
Echinacea tea	Shortens the duration of a cold
Ginger tea	Helps relieve stomach upset or nausea associated with a cold
Elderberry tea	Reduces symptoms of a cold

Safety Smarts: Vitamin C: If you take too much, it can cause gastrointestinal problems. Echinacea: Do not use if you have leukemia (it raises white blood cell counts).

FEVER SMARTS WITH DR. CHILDS

MARC CHILDS, M.D.

Dr. Marc Childs, a pediatrician, takes a simple and smart approach when it comes to treating children with a fever. That means he is, for the most part, anti-medication for fevers, colds and coughs.

Parents have a fever phobia, according to Dr. Childs. "All a fever tells you is that your immune system has been turned on like a warning light. And it's not necessarily a harmful thing. A fever is a normal part of your immune system and it helps your immune system to function properly. So fever is actually a good thing."

Here are some common fever facts and myths, according to Dr. Childs, that you should be aware of.

- *Fact: Normal temperature ranges in children from 97.5°F to 100.3°F.* However, 100.4°F is considered a fever.
- *Fact: Beware if your child looks sick regardless of a fever.* If your child is not responding, is having difficulty breathing, is not talking or walking normally, or has any altered state of consciousness, consult with your doctor immediately.
- *Fact: Steer clear of baby aspirin for kids.* Baby aspirin is no longer recommended for children because of the risk of Reye's syndrome. Aspirin should never be used for children except under the direct supervision of a physician.
- *Fact: Putting a child in a cold bath is foolish.* If you want to put them in a warm bath that's fine, but do not wrap them in cold towels.
- *Myth: A fever means that you have a serious infection.* That is absolutely not true. In children under the age of 8 weeks, it means that they potentially have a serious infection and that is a completely different approach and they should be hospitalized. If a child is vaccinated, and they are between 8 weeks and 3 years, their risk of having a serious infection

with a high fever is probably less than 10 percent (it's much lower if the child is over the age of 3).

- *Myth: Fevers cause seizures.* That is absolutely not true. Note, however, that fevers can cause seizures in children who are predisposed to seizure.
- *Myth: Fevers cause brain damage.* That is not true—unless it gets to 108°F. The only children who ever get fevers as high as 108°F are those who get meningitis, and that's what causes the brain damage.
- *Myth: Rush your child to the emergency room if he or she has a fever.* The best question you can ask parents on the phone is, "If your child didn't have fever would you be as worried?" And if the answer is "No" then you tell them not to worry. If they answer is, 'Yes, I'm really worried,' then that child should be seen," says Dr. Childs.

So how does Dr. Childs treat his kids when they have a fever? "If my children have fever and they're comfortable, they continue to have fever—without any treatment. We give them extra fluids. If they become uncomfortable or irritable or can't sleep as a result of their fever, then we give them Tylenol to bring their fever down," he says. "Again, you really don't want to treat fever unless you have to, because it helps your immune system to function better."

Doc's Rx to Heal Yourself

- Drink water and herbal tea to flush toxins out of the body.
- Wash your hands frequently to safeguard yourself from contracting a cold or flu from a contagious person.
- If you feel as though you're coming down with a cold, take vitamin C, echinacea, and zinc.
- Exercise daily to build up your immune system.
- Practice destressing techniques to keep your stress levels down and immune defenses up.

BIOS

Marc Childs, M.D., is a 36-year-old attending pediatrician at the Mount Kisco Medical Group in Brewster, New York, and an assistant professor of pediatrics at New York Medical College. He received his M.D. at Case Western Reserve University. He is married, has two children, and lives in Chappaqua, New York.

Ray Sahelian, M.D., obtained a bachelor of science degree in nutrition from Drexel University and completed his doctoral training at Thomas Jefferson Medical School, both in Philadelphia. He is certified by the American Board of Family Practice. He is also a popular and respected physician and medical writer. He is the author of *Mind Boosters* (St. Martin's). Dr. Sahelian, at 43, is single and is in private practice in Marina Del Rey, California, where he also lives. Web site:http:// www.raysahelian.com.

13

Fatigue and Fibromyalgia

DR. CONLEY'S ENERGIZING REGIMEN

EDWARD CONLEY, D.O.

Ever mumble, "I am so tired," or, "I don't have any energy"? Well, according to Dr. Edward Conley, who has treated thousands of patients with chronic fatigue syndrome and fibromyalgia (another debilitating condition), you're not alone. According to him, an estimated 80 percent of adults complain of fatigue at one time or another.

"If you told me to walk up to somebody on the street and try to ascertain what sort of health they were in by asking two questions, one would be 'How is your energy?' and the other, 'How is your sex drive?' And if they said, 'My energy is fine and my sex drive is great,' then I could walk away from them about 80 percent sure that they were in good health," points out Dr. Conley.

"Most doctors don't understand how interconnected we are," says Dr. Conley, who knows that if your energy is low it will affect your brain function, immunity, detoxification, muscle strength, and sexual health. Dr. Conley works with all levels of fatigue. In fact, he told me that he has been known to work 60- to 80-hour weeks. Therefore, he fuels his body to prevent fatigue.

"Chronic stress can interfere with sleep, wear down the adrenal glands (especially if your diet has been suboptimal), and produce adrenaline, which causes free radical damage to our energy machinery," explains Dr. Conley.

He adds, "Nutrition is vital. The Krebs cycle [one of the primary biochemical cycles in our body where you burn fat and sugar to be converted to energy] must have minerals, vitamins (especially the B complex), cofactors (like CoQ_{10}), and essential amino acids to run efficiently. Any deficiency will slow energy and therefore everything else (like immunity and brain function), since everything runs on energy."

Also vital is exercise. "If you are in normal health, conditioning will slowly help your energy. I do a walking program, or treadmill or stairstep, and weight lifting," says Dr. Conley. "I want to stress, however, that if someone has CFS they can't exercise their way out of it; indeed, aerobic exercise will usually make them worse. This is another important difference between regular fatigue and CFS."

DOCTOR'S LINGO

Chronic fatigue syndrome (CFS): Now also called chronic fatigue immune dysfunction syndrome (CFIDS), is a disease where someone has profound fatigue all of the time, according to Dr. Conley. He estimates that 10 million people suffer from CFS. This fatigue is so severe that it makes it hard to work or to function in home life. Some people are so severely affected that they can't cook, clean, or take a shower! Many of course can't work. It does not go away with rest. Being overworked or tired occasionally goes away with rest.

SUCCESS STORY

Dr. Conley's most unforgettable patient, Debbie, at 23, was so ill that when he first saw her he thought that she had AIDS (acquired immunodeficiency syndrome). "She was wasted to 82 pounds and couldn't eat very well. She had infection after infection and, of course, couldn't work (she was a reporter)."

The treatment: It was a very extensive program; however, some of the things Dr. Conley did to help this woman corrected all her vitamin, mineral, amino acid, and antioxidant deficiencies. This allowed her Krebs cycle energy to improve, which also improved her immune function. "It took a lot of hard work and insight, but it was worth all the effort. Now she is a reporter for a Michigan newspaper, is married with children, and in good health."

THE DOC'S SUPPLEMENT LIST

These following nutrients are what Dr. Conley prescribes to his patients (and takes himself, except NADH, which is more for treatment) who are having energy problems.

Supplement	What It Does
NADH	The energizing coenzyme NADH (nicotinamide adenine dinucleotide) stimulates cellular production of the neurotransmitters dopamine, noradrenaline, and serotonin; it enhances cognitive and memory functions
CoQ_{10}	This fat-soluble compound acts as an antioxidant that can boost energy production in nearly every cell in the body; lowers fatigue
B vitamins	B vitamins are cofactors in numerous reactions in the body, including energy production
Essential amino acids	Help the body to run efficiently

Multivitamin-and-mineral supplement	Ensures that you get vitamins and minerals that you may be lacking in your daily diet, which are important for energy production
Vitamin C	It's an immune enhancer antioxidant to help stave off colds, muscle strength, which can zap your energy

Safety Smarts: Vitamin C: If you take too much, it can cause gastrointestinal problems.

SHAKING THE ACHES AND PAINS WITH DR. PODELL

RICHARD PODELL, M.D.

Several years ago I wrote an article entitled "Shaking the Aches" in which I learned that sufferers of chronic pain and fatigue could have undiagnosed fibrositis, sometimes called fibromyalgia. Recently, I watched an episode of the television series *Strong Medicine* in which a young woman was finally diagnosed with this difficult-to-pinpoint pain syndrome.

Fibromyalgia means "pain in the muscles." It's characterized by tenderness with pressure in 11 or more of 18 "tender points," explains Dr. Richard Podell, who told me he has the tender points but doesn't have the aches. About 50 percent of his patients have fibromyalgia or chronic fatigue syndrome and are learning how to cope with chronic aches and pains, often in the back of the neck, low back, and lateral hips.

According to Dr. Podell, "These people are vulnerable to stress, although it's very hard to tell whether they were that way before they got sick or since they got sick. So the stress and anxiety is the secondary part of being in pain and not sleeping well."

Dr. Podell recommends that his fibromyalgia patients follow a basic program that includes the following:

- *Adequate sleep.* "One of the complaints you see in almost everyone suffering from fibromyalgia is that they wake up feeling tired, as if they haven't slept, even if they have slept," explains Dr. Podell. He works on helping his patients get proper sleep hygiene such as the scheduling of sleep, the comfort of the bedroom, the habits of getting ready to go to sleep. He combines recommending good sleep habits with either herbal or prescription sleep aids. "The best ones are the low-dose antidepressants used for sleep—not depression. This can help fibromyalgia in about half of the patients within a couple of days."

- *Exercise.* Aerobic exercise (such as walking) can improve the symptoms of fibrositis, including sleep disturbances, fatigue, and pain. "Do the right amount of exercise: not too much, not too little," points out Dr. Podell. "If you don't do any exercise you're going to get worse." In addition, muscles need a chance to relax, which can be done by muscle stretching, muscle fitness, massage, heat, cold, and liniments.

- *Diet.* "I put fibromyalgia patients on a basic nutritional program, which is low sugar, no alcohol. Reducing caffeine if they're addicted to it," says Dr. Podell. He also recommends five servings a day of fruits and vegetables, which are antioxidant-rich and can boost the immune system.

FACTS F.Y.I.

According to Dr. Podell:

- Fibrositis most often strikes women between ages 20 and 50.
- The most common complaints are chronic aches and pains in the back of the neck, low back, and lateral hips.
- About 75 percent of people also experience sleep disturbances, which explains why an estimated 80 percent battle ongoing fatigue, and there are probably other causes as well.

SUCCESS STORY

Dr. Podell recalls one woman, a single journalist. At 32, Sally who had been suffering chronic pain and fatigue for about eight years. "Most of the doctors said it was all in her head. One of them said she had lupus [a life-threatening autoimmune disease], but it turned out that she didn't."

The fact was, Sally was very angry and frustrated because she couldn't do what she wanted to do: simply work and play. "But because of the aches, fatigue, poor sleep, irritable bowel, and headaches, she couldn't concentrate well enough or have the physical stamina to reliably work day by day," says Dr. Podell, who helped this woman get back her life.

"First, I made sure that she wasn't in fact depressed. She was enthusiastic about doing things. The problem was, whenever she did anything, the next day she crashed and got more tired, more foggy in the head, and more achy," recalls Dr. Podell.

The plan: He put her on a slow-motion exercise plan, which meant she increased exercise very slowly. She got off coffee, alcohol, and sugar. She began to eat lots of antioxidant-rich fruits and vegetables. She was also given plenty of magnesium. One year later, Sally was back on the job.

THE DOC'S SUPPLEMENT LIST

Here are some of the supplements that Dr. Podell recommends to his fibromyalgia patients.

Supplement	What It Does
Magnesium	Mineral that can help muscle pain and stress
Vitamin-and-mineral supplement	Vital for proper functioning of biochemical enzymes, which allows the function of the biochemical pathways

Essentail fatty acids	Rich in fatty acids, omega-3s and omega-6s, which can support the entire body's system
N-acetyl cysteine	It is a precursor to glutathione, an antioxidant that is important for energy production; boosts the immune system

Safety Smarts: Omega oils: Don't take high doses of fish oil capsules if you are taking NSAIDs (nonsteroidal anti-inflammatory drugs). It may increase gastrointestinal ulcers and bleeding.

DOC'S RX TO HEAL YOURSELF

- Take NADH to enhance your cognitive and memory function.
- Use CoQ_{10} to boost energy levels.
- Take a multivitamin-and-mineral to get adequate vitamins and minerals.
- Take vitamin C to enhance immunity so you don't get sick, which can zap energy.
- Learn good sleep hygiene.
- Chill out because stress and anxiety can zap your energy production.
- Eat smart for energy.
- Consider taking energy-boosting nutrients—magnesium, a vitamin-mineral supplement, fish oils, evening primrose oil, and N-acetyl cysteine.

BIOS

Edward Conley, D.O., has a Fatigue and Fibromyalgic Clinic in Flint, Michigan. He graduated from Michigan State University in East Lansing. He is the author of *America Exhausted* (Vitality

Press). At 45, he is single and resides in Grand Blanc, Michigan. Web site: www.cfids.com.

Richard Podell, M.D., is a doctor who practices integrative medicine. He received his M.D. at Harvard University in Boston, Massachusetts. Dr. Podell is the director of the Podell Medical Center in New Providence, New Jersey. He is the author of *Doctor, Why Am I Always So Tired?* (Pharos Books) and is professor of family medicine at the Robert Wood Johnson Medical School in New Brunswick. At 58, he is married and has three children.

14

Immunity

Dr. Rosenbaum's Nutritional Regimen

MICHAEL E. ROSENBAUM, M.D.

84

Did you know that your body is ready to go to war? It is. In fact, it's on alert from the time you're born until the day you die. The enemies are viral and bacterial invaders that are threatening your health. Although you may not be aware of a potential battle going on, there are things you can do to stay healthy and keep the peace.

The answer lies in the immune system. The immune system—that is, your body's defense system, made up of billions of white blood cells or "warriors" that are ready to destroy potential enemies—can protect you against illness if it's fed the right foods.

Dr. Michael Rosenbaum, coauthor of *Super Supplements* (Penguin), made it quite clear he is savvy when it comes to the immune system. Most of his patients have immune-related illnesses from allergies, chronic fatigue syndrome, or fibromyalgia, and he is also called an environmental physician, so he works a lot with the effect of chemicals on the immune response.

"The word *immune* means freedom from taxes and it's an old Latin expression. It's your body's way of freeing you from the taxation of being burdened by microbes that are trying to destroy you," explains Dr. Rosenbaum.

"The immune system is responsible for what goes on in the body. It is vitally connected to all parts of our body. We now know that heart disease, for instance, may be caused by infection and by inflammation and immune processes. That immune cells may be partially a cause of heart disease. So many of the degenerative diseases like arthritis, cancer, and heart disease are vitally connected to immune health, and even depression, anxiety, and lack of sleep have a profound effect on the immune system," he adds.

Doctor's Lingo

Lymphocytes: Your first line of defense against invading bacteria and viruses is the skin and mucous membranes of your body. The second kind of defense is these white blood cells called lymphoctyes, which track down germs and destroy them like little Pacmen. Lymphocytes are made in the bone marrow and stored in the lymph, fluid that flows throughout the body. Two different types of lymphocytes circulate: B-cells and T-cells.

B-cells: Lymphocytes stay in the bone marrow until they reach maturity. Then they circulate in the bloodstream and end up in the lymph systems and organs such as the spleen, tonsils, and adenoids. B-cells make and release certain proteins, called antibodies, that identify and destroy invaders.

T-cells: The other type of lymphocytes, T-cells leave the bone marrow early in their life cycle and move to the thymus gland. Later, the T-cells, like the B-cells, enter the bloodstream and end up in the tonsils and spleen. These cells consist of helper T-cells working with the B-cells; killer T-cells, which make deadly substances to kill invaders; and suppressor T-cells, which keep the immune system working efficiently.

Macrophages: These cells are often called scavenger or antigen-presenting cells because they detect foreign invaders and alert T-cells and B-cells to their presence.

(Source: Cal Orey, "Immunity Nutrition," *Energy Times*, September 2000, page 26)

DIET AND IMMUNITY

"The immune system is more dependent on nutrition status than perhaps any other organ system in the body. And the reason is that it has such a dynamic rapid turnover of cells. Any system in the body that turns over so rapidly is extremely dependent on nutrition status," says Dr. Rosenbaum.

There are two things in the diet to be careful about: the sugar content and the fat content. Both high-fat diets and sugar tend to suppress the immune response, says Dr. Rosenbaum. And even more important than eating a nutrient-dense diet, these two culprits should be avoided for maintaining a strong immune system.

While Dr. Rosenbaum tries to eat a nutrient-rich diet, which can strengthen the immune system, like most of us, he is only human and may not eat as well as he'd like every day. Therefore, he supplements his diet "quite richly."

THE DOC'S SUPPLEMENT LIST

These are some of the supplements Dr. Rosenbaum turns to that help keep his immune system strong and healthy.

Supplement	What It Does
Green tea	Rich in antioxidants, which help to stall immune decline by neutralizing the disease-causing molecules called free radicals
Multivitamin-and-mineral richly endowed with vitamins C and E, selenium, and beta carotene	C helps supercharge your immune system; E, another antioxidant, can help guard against environmental toxins, stimulate the immune response, and guard against life-threatening infections; carotene strengthens the immune system

Carotenoids	Antioxidants (lutein and lycopene), which boost the immune system, aid indirectly in the response of T-cells and B-cells

DOC'S RX TO HEAL YOURSELF

- Eat a nutrient-rich diet to bolster your immune system.
- Drink green tea, which can forestall immune decline and help neutralize disease-causing free radicals.
- Take a multivitamin-and-mineral supplement that includes immune-boosting antioxidant vitamin C, vitamin E, and selenium, and don't forget beta carotene and carotenoids to boost immunity, too.

BIO

Michael E. Rosenbaum, M.D., has a private practice in Corte Medera, California. He graduated from the Albert Einstein College of Medicine in New York City. He is the coauthor of *Solving the Puzzle of Chronic Fatigue Syndrome* (Life Sciences Press). He is 59, has two children, and lives in Corte Medera.

PART IV

Bones, Joints, and Muscles

About ten years ago, I loved being a new dog owner. I jogged with my Brittany at the free-run dog park, explored landscaped man-made ponds, and ran him on a leash through the suburbs. But one day, after a dog-on-leash run during which Dylan had pulled too hard and fast, my lower back hurt so much that I yowled like a pup in pain.

After a visit to a local chiropractor, I learned that I was suffering from sciatica, a pain felt down the back and outer side of my thigh and leg. The attack had been brought on by Dylan's pulling on his leash. After a few chiropractic treatments, ice packs, and bed rest I was fine. However it was a wake-up call to start exercising and change my diet.

All-too-common pains and aches like those I experienced can occur for many reasons. Part IV, "Bones, Joints, and Muscles," is about the incredible power of bones, joints, and muscles. The power of the spine is not some mysterious thing. Your bones, joints, and muscles are key to maintaining the ability to move and stay active at any age.

Dr. John Hardesty Bland, renowned rheumatologist and author of *Live Long, Die Fast* (Fairview Press), declares that stretching is the key to fighting arthritis.

Elsewhere, Dr. Alan Pressman advocates good nutrition for

our bones, joints, and muscles. "If your diet is inadequate in calories or protein, vitamins or minerals or fats and carbohydrates, your body does not have the fuel to support normal healthy growth and tissue repair," he explains. Improper nutrition will wreak havoc on your total body because your bones are the pillars of your support, which depend upon a steady intake of nutrients.

Drs. Arthur Brownstein and David Schechter know that prevention and treatment of back pain is a body, mind, and spirit experience. And orthopedic surgeon Dr. Irwin Siegel, M.D.'s practical advice can help stave off kids' bone injuries.

Melba Iris Ovalle, M.D., and Alan Gaby, M.D., are each aware of the importance of ways to stop (and even reverse) the crippling effects of bone loss. And both doctors tell you how women and men can fight back at any age.

On the following pages the doctors will share valuable information gathered from their personal experience, clinics, and case histories. Included are tips on using diet, vitamins and minerals, and lifestyle changes. These experts will tell you how to save your bones, joints, and muscles and fight aches and pains.

15

Arthritis

DR. PRESSMAN'S ANTI-ARTHRITIS TREATMENT

ALAN PRESSMAN, D.C.

Like many other doctors, Dr. Alan Pressman sees countless patients who suffer from arthritis aches and pains. He tells me that he treats his patients (about 60 percent have arthritis; they are both men and women, mostly age 50 and over) with chiropractic methods and good nutrition.

I asked Dr. Pressman whether he actually does chiropractic on people who have arthritis. "Sure," he told me. "What happens in the arthritic patient is that the joint itself starts to degenerate. There's a dehydration of the cartilage, the range of motion of the joints degenerates, and instead of bone rubbing on cartilage, which is a very smooth surface, you've got bone rubbing on bone.

"One of the examples I use all of the time," adds Dr. Pressman, "is that if you took two ice cubes out of the freezer and wet them and rubbed them together, that's how smoothly a joint should move. There's evidence to show that joint fluid is eight times more fluid than two ice cubes rubbing together. In arthritis, especially degenerative arthritis or degenerative joint disease, the joint dries up and you've got bone rubbing on bone. And that is what causes the dramatic [decrease in] range of motion."

He continues, "What's done in chiropractic is to put those joints into proper alignment, reestablishing normal range of motion." And millions of people may benefit from Dr. Pressman's "joint efforts," since this many fall victim to arthritis according to the statistics.

FACTS F.Y.I.

According to the Arthritis Foundation:

- Osteoarthritis affects nearly 21 million Americans, mostly after age 45; women are more commonly affected than men.
- Rheumatoid arthritis affects 2.1 million Americans, mostly women.
- 1.5 million women have rheumatoid arthritis compared to 600,000 men.

BONE BUILDERS

"Any nutrient that strengthens bone, reduces inflammation, and increases the fluidity of the joint will be successful in managing the arthritic patient," points out Dr. Pressman.

"In the arthritic patient, *just* doing nutritional care is totally inadequate. In other words, if you're going to take all of the nutrients [listed in "The Doc's Supplement List" on page 125], nothing is going to be successful until those joints are put into motion. Because the only way joints can get nourished is if they are in motion because they do not have a direct blood supply," he adds.

The ultimate solution: It's the combination of nonforced chiropractic technique, adequate nutrition, supplements, and exercise that is the arthritis answer, says Dr. Pressman.

Success Story

Dr. Pressman recalls a fifty-something male former world light heavyweight champion boxer who had arthritis to the point where he couldn't work out anymore. The combination of physical manipulation—exercise is crucial—and a nutritional regime enabled him to go back to the gym.

Tony saw Dr. Pressman twice a week for about three months. He took fish oil supplements, two to three fish meals per week, resveratrol, proanthocyanidin, and glucosamine. He was very determined and stuck to the program. The outcome: The champ is back at the gym, and he has good range of motion with minimal to no pain.

THE DOC'S SUPPLEMENT LIST

Here are several supplements that Dr. Pressman recommends to his patients who suffer from arthritis.

Supplement	What It Does
Glucosamine	Recommended for anyone who has joint pain inflammation. It's a substance that your body makes. It has the ability to repair the tissues of bone, ligament, and cartilage. It also may help rebuild bone, reduce inflammation, and relieve pain.
Proanthocyanidin	It's an antioxidant, a flavonoid that comes commonly from grape seed. It appears to have a mild anti-inflammatory effect.
Resveratrol	Another substance that comes from grape seed, which is a natural inhibitor of what we call a pro-inflammatory enzyme.

Vitamin C	This antioxidant vitamin is necessary to build bone.
Boron, vitamin D, phosphorus	All of these minerals are involved in the synthesis of bone. Calcium appears to migrate from inside the bone to outside the bone, resulting in inflammation and calcification of the joints.
Extract of philodendron	This comes from extract of the philodendron house plant. There is a fairly new combination of philodendron and resveratrol from grape seed that is a phenomenal anti-inflammatory.
Omega-3 oils	It is important for lubrication of joints; it also reduces pro-inflammatory chemicals called prostaglandins.

Safety Smarts: Vitamin C: If you take too much, it can cause gastrointestinal problems. Omega-3 oils: Don't take high doses of fish oil capsules if you are taking NSAIDs (nonsteroidal anti-inflammatory drugs). It may increase gastrointestinal ulcers and bleeding.

SECOND OPINION: DR. BLAND'S STAY-ACTIVE PLAN

JOHN HARDESTY BLAND, M.D.

John Hardesty Bland, M.D., never tries to hide that he's over 80 or a geriatric jock. He proudly declares that he is active in walking—not bingo or shuffleboard.

The world-renowned rheumatologist tackles the aches and pains of joints in an active anti-arthritis style. His secret for preventing arthritis is not the tired tradition of taking it easy and slowing down. It's a "Don't act your age" attitude, he insists. In fact, Bland stays a kid at heart and defies arthritis by keeping flexible with exercise.

Some research suggests that gentle stretching exercises, such as yoga may indeed provide relief for osteoarthritis of the hands, relieve anxiety, reduce depression, and create a sense of well-being. More research is needed.

Dr. Bland performs daily morning stretching exercises (24 exercises, 24 minutes), weekly walks (10 hours), and running-jogging sessions (2½ to 3 hours).

Dr. Bland's Ten Stretching Exercises

Here are ten stretching exercises to help get you started on Dr. Bland's Stay-Active plan.

- *Exercise 1.* Seated on the floor, grasp your right knee with your right hand. With your left hand, pull your right leg as far back as is comfortable. Hold this position for 20 seconds. Repeat on the opposite side.
- *Exercise 2.* Flex your head and neck, keeping your chin on your chest. Lock your knees. Bend at the waist, reaching for the floor as far as you comfortably can. Hold this for 20 seconds.
- *Exercise 3.* Standing erect, reach forward, stretching as far as you can. Hold for 20 seconds.
- *Exercise 4.* Lock your knees in the straight position, holding the thigh muscles tight. Look up toward the ceiling. Extend your neck, arching your back and neck as far as possible, straining to extend your entire spine. Hold both arms to the rear as far as you can. Hold for 20 seconds.
- *Exercise 5.* Stand erect, with your right arm straight at your side. Reach behind your back and grasp your right wrist with your left hand. Lift your right forearm as nearly parallel to the floor as possible. Hold for 20 seconds. Repeat on the opposite side.
- *Exercise 6.* Spread your legs as far apart as possible; then reach for the floor. Hold for 20 seconds, stretching the inside of both thighs—a stretch you can feel.

- *Exercise 7.* Standing in your best posture, chin up, keeping your arms straight by your side, slowly rotate your right shoulder, making as complete a circle as possible in as nearly vertical a plane as possible. Make as big a circle as you can, stretching all the way. Repeat 20 times. Perform the same rotation sequence on the opposite side.
- *Exercise 8.* Standing, extend both arms straight out from your sides. You will find that with your palms facing the floor, you cannot bring palms together over your head. Raise your arms as high as you can and hold this position for a count of 20. Rotate your arms and you'll find you can bring your palms together above your head. Hold for 20 seconds.
- *Exercise 9.* Standing on one foot and, if necessary using a wall or post to help you balance, grasp your right foot at about your toe level (forefoot) and bring your heel up to your buttock, stretching passively as much as is comfortable. Hold for 20 seconds. Repeat the procedure on the opposite side.
- *Exercise 10.* Standing with feet at least 12 inches apart and about 3 inches from a counter, put both hands down on the counter or other stable surface. With your feet and toes as far back as possible, lean forward, holding your legs straight, stretching the back of your calves as much as possible. Hold for 20 seconds.

DOC'S RX TO HEAL YOURSELF

- Opt for natural anti-inflamatories such as glucosamine, proanthocyanidin, resveratrol, and extract of philodendron.
- Try bone aids such as vitamins C and D and minerals boron and phosphorus.
- Use omega-3 supplements to help lubricate joints and lessen inflammation.
- Do daily stretches to provide physical and mental relief of arthritis-related problems.

Bios

John Hardesty Bland, M.D., is a professor emeritus at the University of Vermont College of Medicine. He's written ten books including *The Complete Mall Walker's Handbook: Walking for Fun and Fitness* (Fairview Press). He has been married for 55 years. The Blands live where they raised their family, in Pleasant Valley, Cambridge, Vermont. He is an octogenarian with four children and ten grandchildren.

Alan Pressman, D.C., Ph.D., is a chiropractor and board-certified dietitian/nutritionist, and is the host of the radio program *Healthline with Dr. Pressman,* which brings health information to millions of people. He attended the Chiropractic Institute of New York. At 58, he is the author of various books on alternative care including *Integrative Medicine* (St. Martin's Press), *The Complete Idiot's Guide to Vitamins and Minerals* (Hungry Minds) and *The Complete Idiot's Guide to Alternative Medicine* (Alpha Books). He is the director of the Magaziner Center for Wellness and Anti-Aging Medicine in Cherry Hill, New Jersey, where natural non-toxic therapies are emphasized. He resides in New York City, is married, and has two children. Web site: www.DrPressman.com.

16

Back Pain

Q & A WITH DR. BROWNSTEIN

ARTHUR BROWNSTEIN, M.D.

Dr. Arthur Brownstein endured 20 years of debilitating back pain—before and after surgery. But the doctor told me that he has ended up a healthier and happier person thanks to his self-healing efforts.

He is hardly alone. "Back pain is an epidemic. It's crippling our workforce and costing Americans $100 billion a year in work-related disability, doctor visits, treatments, and surgery," points out Dr. Brownstein in his book *Healing Back Pain Naturally* (Harbor Press).

However, this doctor got rid of his pain in the back. Here, read on and see exactly how the physician healed himself, naturally.

Q. *Please explain your personal bout with back pain.*
A. I had recurrent, disabling back pain with a diagnosis of degenerative disc disease (in which the cartilage shock absorbers in between the vertebrae start to degenerate from wear and tear and start to collapse) at the very young age of 27.

Q. *Did it get worse?*
A. When I was 36 I ruptured a disc and I ended up on an operating table and went through surgery. The surgery was supposed to help me get better, and it did to a point. It decompressed the nerve. My whole leg was numb from the ruptured disc. But I ended up with a gaping hole in my back because they had to cut through two bones to get to the disc and then those bones were thrown in the garbage can and just muscle was sewed over the hole. So it left me with a huge hole in my back and weakened. For three years I floundered. I was a chronic pain patient.

Q. *So what did you do for the pain?*
A. I was addicted to pain pills. I was depressed. I was suicidal. After three years of not getting anywhere (I couldn't work as a doctor because I couldn't even stand up without the pain), I was offered a second operation that included spinal fusion, bone grafting, and metal plates and screws. I refused that and left the country.

I ended up in India, studying yoga and mind-body techniques and looking at a more holistic approach. I found information that was never taught to me in medical school, information that very few Western doctors were focusing on. I got better.

Q. *In your book* Healing Back Pain Naturally *you mention that vitamin deficiencies are linked to disease in the spine. Does that pertain to your case?*
A. No. Vitamin deficiencies are not that common for spine problems. But you need to be aware of the possibility that they exist. I'm not a supplement person. I used to supplement many years ago. Once in a while I will take some St. John's wort, which is good for your immune system and is recognized in Germany as a mild antidepressant. Sometimes at night I will take a little kava root, which is a muscle relaxer. I really don't take supplements because I'm a vegetarian, so I eat a well-rounded diet full of fruits and vegetables and whole grains to make sure I get most of my vitamins.

Q. *What's your personal Rx to keep your back healthy?*
A. The things I do to keep it healthy are focus on the muscles and

make sure that I don't overload my back. I practice relaxation, recognizing the role that the mind plays in the back. I'm always listening to my back. I make sure that I'm sleeping in good positions. I do a lot of stretching and I teach yoga. I'm on the up generally, and when I'm feeling down I process that and don't just ignore it or suppress it. I drink a lot of fluids.

Q. *What is your biggest tip for healing your back naturally?*
A. I look at it holistically, not mechanically. I treat myself as a human being with a mind, body, and spirit. It's the most important thing to do. And if I do feel my back tensing up or getting tight, I usually take an inventory of myself. Have I been sitting at the computer too many hours writing books and slouching and not getting enough exercise? Am I under stress? Am I not drinking enough fluids? Is my diet out of balance?

Q. *Why is the back so important to our well-being?*
A. If you talk to the chiropractors they'll tell you that the spine is the center of your nervous system—your most important electrical neurological conduit in your body that communicates from your brain to the rest of your body. And when your spine is healthy, then the nerves that come out of the spine are optimally functioning so that every organ and system in your body is positively influenced.

Q. *Do you see patients with back problems, and do you try to get them to think of healing the back in a holistic way as you did?*
A. Absolutely. I want to remind people that we are not just machines. There's a lot more to us than the mechanical aspect. My back problem ended up being a gift. Going through chronic pain, understanding the deeper mystical value of pain, is a way of getting your attention to areas of deeper, emotional pain that you might have successfully suppressed.

And when you're not at peace with yourself, loving yourself, you're out of balance. And if your life is out of balance, those factors come into your back and throw your back out of balance. If you still don't get the message, then you can try all the exterior means of healing that you want—but at some point you're going to have to turn inward to the vast universe of inner resources that your body possesses.

FACTS F.Y.I.

According to Back Care, the U.K. Charity National Organization for Healthy Backs:

- Women's back pain tends to last longer than men's. Men are more apt to have a short, sharp attack.
- Women are more likely than men to have restricted activity due to back pain.
- Menstrual periods can trigger back pain.
- Studies in the United States indicate that about one-half of pregnant women get back pain.
- Men's back pain is often the result of an injury; women's pain occurs as a result of conditions or activities in their everyday lives, including domestic work and child care.
- The main triggers for women's back pain at home are carrying heavy objects, gardening, and vacuuming.

THE DOC'S SUPPLEMENT LIST

While Dr. Brownstein currently is not a supplement person since he eats a nutrient-dense diet, in his book *Healing Back Pain Naturally*, he does recommend getting adequate daily amounts of the following nutrients, and he takes St. John's wort occasionally himself.

Supplement	What It Does
Calcium	A lack of the mineral calcium may show up in your spine as osteoporosis, which can lead to spinal fractures and back pain

Vitamin B$_{12}$	Insufficient vitamin B$_{12}$ can cause back pain and degeneration of nerve cells in the spinal cord
Vitamin D	A deficiency of vitamin D can result in rickets, a condition that can cause severe deformities in the spine, especially in childhood
Vitamin E	This antioxidant vitamin helps to repair damaged muscle tissue in the back
Kava	An herb that helps to relax muscles
St. John's wort	An antidepressant herbal remedy

Safety Smarts: St. John's wort may cause sun sensitivity. Do not mix with other antidepressants.

PREVENTING SPORTS INJURIES WITH DR. SCHECHTER

DAVID SCHECHTER, M.D.

Ever wonder what doctors personally do to prevent sports injuries? According to Dr. David Schechter, these ten basic tips are what he follows himself and recommends to his patients.

1. Get exercise regularly. Find something you enjoy and make that your activity. It doesn't matter what it is, if you enjoy it you're going to do it more regularly.
2. Warm up with a walk, a light jog, or a slower version of the activity you're going to do—every time. And easy does it. Remember, stretching should be done gently.
3. If you get injured, use *ice. Ice, ice, ice.* Ten or 15 minutes is usually about right, then rest and repeat. Too many people use heat inappropriately.
4. If you're worried about injury or you're fatigued, that's

when you get hurt. Don't exercise when you're exhausted. Destress before you push yourself hard.

5. If you get injured, use ice, then start walking or doing activities slowly to get back into things. Try not to worry. Most injuries heal. If you're hurting a lot or can't move, see a doctor.

6. A few days of anti-inflammatories (such as ibuprofen) are a wonderful way to help the body to start healing. However, a few months of these medications should only be taken under careful medical supervision to preserve your kidneys and liver.

7. Worrying too much about your injuries, especially back and neck aches, is a sure way to have them continue or become chronic. Think positively and leave your stress at the door.

8. Eat regularly. Eat a moderately low-fat diet with some vegetables of varying colors and eat fairly low on the food chain.

9. The best equipment isn't always necessary, but buy good equipment that fits you properly and keep it well maintained.

10. Sometimes the easiest cure for an overuse injury to the legs is to buy a new pair of sneakers. And it's cheaper than an office visit or an X-ray.

DR. JENKINS'S ESSENTIAL NUTRIENT

KEVIN D. JENKINS, D.C.

Check out the film *Cast Away*. Actor Tom Hanks shows us quickly that water intake is top priority to stay alive. And in real life water is nothing to take lightly either, according to Dr. Kevin Jenkins, a chiropractor.

The human body is made up of about 75 percent water. Water keeps the body running, and indeed, says Dr. Jenkins, you will not survive as long without water as you will without food.

No doubt, water is this doctor's favorite nutrient. "Without water I feel like an old man," he says. And for good reason. After all, water keeps him (and you) alive, flushes toxins from your body, boosts energy levels, and helps to keep you regular.

Adds Dr. Jenkins: "Here's another thing to think about. When you go to bed at night you're a half inch shorter than when you wake up. If the body is not properly hydrated, the discs in the spine will be the last parts of the body to get water. So you can begin the degenerative process by losing a thousandth of an inch throughout your entire spine a day if you're not properly hydrated."

Dr. Jenkins prefers pure mountain spring water because too many of the others have been filtered or have chemical additives that are causing their own host of problems. He drinks a whopping sixteen 8-ounce glasses (at least) of water daily. "I wake up in the morning and drink a quart of water the first thing. I feel better when I do that. I do martial arts, and when I don't get enough water the next morning I feel arthritic because my body has not been able to flush the toxins out of the body." But note that while he drinks mega amounts of water, he recommends that the average person should drink a minimum of eight 8-ounce glasses per day.

DOC'S RX TO HEAL YOURSELF

- If you are depressed because of back pain, try St. John's wort, which is a mild antidepressant.
- Use kava to help relax your muscles.
- Practice relaxation techniques to relax your total body.
- Treat your back holistically: mind, body, and spirit.
- Learn how to find peace and balance in your life.
- Opt for spine strengtheners such as vitamin B_{12}, vitamin D, and calcium.
- And don't forget antioxidant E to help restore pain-damaged muscle tissue in the back.
- Exercise regularly.

- Eat a low-fat diet.
- If you get injured use *ice*.
- Use the right equipment to avoid injuries.
- Be sure to drink at least eight 8-ounce glasses of water (preferably mountain spring water) daily.

Bios

Arthur Brownstein, M.D., is board certified in preventive medicine. He attended Jefferson Medical College in Philadelphia. He is an assistant clinical professor of medicine at the University of Hawaii and also works at his Princeville Medical Clinic in Princeville, Hawaii. At 51, he is married and has a 3-year-old son.

Kevin D. Jenkins, D.C., is a chiropractor and is licensed in homeopathy. He received his degree from Palmer College of Chiropractic in Davenport, Iowa. His practice is entitled Nevada Integrated Chiropractic in Las Vegas, Nevada. He is 32, is married, has three children, and lives in Las Vegas.

David Schechter, M.D., is on the faculty of the University of Southern California School of Medicine. Dr. Schechter is a board-certified family practice/sports medicine physician who has a clinical practice at the International Orthopedic Center for Joint Disorders in Beverly Hills, California, and is the author of *The Mindbody Workbook* (MindBody Medicine Publications). He is 41 and lives in Los Angeles, California, with his wife and one son 2 years of age. Web site: www.mindbodymedicine.com.

17

Osteoporosis

BEATING BONE LOSS WITH DR. OVALLE

MELBA IRIS OVALLE, M.D.

Dr. Melba Iris Ovalle candidly shares her secondhand experience about how bone loss has touched her life:

> My mother has osteoporosis. She is 72 years old. I watched her go from 5 feet 0 inches to 4 feet 11 inches. She has fractured her wrist, ribs, facial bones, and numerous vertebrae. Worst of all, she is frail and has lost weight. She continues to manifest bone loss by intermittently losing teeth. They are brittle and tend to break off with any food that requires vigorous chewing. As a result, she is afraid to eat and weighs a mere 79 pounds.
>
> Doctors failed to address this problem, which, thinking back now, began when she was just 50 years old. At that time she was in menopause and no hormones were ever given. Furthermore, that was the time she sustained her first fracture after falling off the kitchen stool. My fear is that I will follow in her footsteps. We are both small-framed, thin-boned females.

While in college, I watched in dismay as my mother changed from a physically vibrant and active female to a frail, anxious, and fragile person. As I entered medical school and began my training, I was keenly interested in bone health and how to prevent osteoporosis. I found knowledge is power and learned that this is one disease that can be altered. I began to gain confidence and relay that knowledge and confidence to my patients.

Currently, at 44, I am the medical director of the ENH Osteoporosis and Metabolic Bone Disease Center in Illinois. I have strong convictions when it comes to women's health issues. In my case, bone health is as critical to me as heart disease or a family history of breast cancer. Ironically, hip fractures are the third leading cause of hospitalizations, after cardiovascular diseases and pneumonias. I see patients every day regarding bone disease—almost 90 percent are osteoporosis patients.

Dr. Ovalle is hardly alone in what she has witnessed. The alarming statistics are proof: According to a National Osteoporosis foundation report in February 2002, the number of folks aged 50 or older estimated to be at risk for bone loss and low bone mass is 44 million in 2002—30 million women and 14 million men.

SUCCESS STORY

"I will never forget a patient, Janet, who was sent to me by her internist," says Dr. Ovalle. "She was a thin, elderly Caucasian female. She reminded me a lot of my mother. She weighed only 90 pounds. She had multiple vertebral fractures and back pain. In short, failure to thrive and severe osteoporosis were the diagnosis. I started an aggressive program of nutritional supplements, calcium, vitamin D, and physical therapy. A bisphosphonate was also added to her regimen." Bisphosphonates are potent agents that block the loss or resorption of bone. The most common ones are etidronate, alendronate, and residonate.

In less than three months, Dr. Ovalle continues, the woman returned to her office in a leather outfit, a miniskirt, and a gorgeous hat. She had gained several pounds and now weighed 116 pounds. She was smiling and happy. The transformation was remarkable. According to Dr. Ovalle, the woman said "she felt alive once more."

DR. OVALLE'S PERSONAL BONE-UP PLAN

Like any mother, Dr. Ovalle wants to set a good example for her children. She has three daughters, ages 16, 14, and 11 years old. And now is the time to begin a strong-bones program, she believes.

- *Dietary guidelines.* As for dietary constraints, we have no soda pop in our house. We have eliminated cookies, snacks, and most refined foods. I have to admit, though, we still buy ice cream. At least, it is a good source of calcium. I haven't started using soy or phytoestrogens yet. I may consider it during menopause.
- *Exercise.* No time for exercise! Gotta run! Maybe tomorrow! These were some of the excuses I used to justify my lack of exercise. My family and I walk at least three to four times per week and lift 5-pound weights in front of our favorite television shows.
- *Bone DEXA.* I definitely will get a central DEXA (bone density test) when I am menopausal, even if that is before I turn 50. I have already obtained a Heel ultrasound (a device that measures bone mass) to see where I was with my bone mass. Fortunately, I had a T score of 0.8 (normal). The National Osteoporosis Foundation (NOF) recommends all patients over the age of 65 be screened. Those who are younger with risk factors may need screening sooner.

STRONG BONES AT ANY AGE

To stop bone problems, Dr. Ovalle recommends the following:

- *If you're in your thirties,* consume adequate amounts of calcium and vitamin D. Consider taking a multivitamin supplement, too. Go easy on the alcohol, don't smoke and lift those barbells.
- *If you're in your forties,* schedule enough time to exercise. Weight-bearing exercise is crucial to maintaining and stimulating bone growth. Maintain adequate intake of calcium and vitamin D.
- *If you're in your fifties,* ask your health practitioner to assess your hormone status and to do a baseline Bone DEXA to measure your bone status. The fifties are the decade during which both men and women lose bone rapidly due to the loss of estrogen and testosterone.
- *If you're in your sixties,* review your medications with your health practitioner. The medications used to treat hypertension, arthritis, and thyroid problems often cause bone loss. You should also consider taking a multivitamin with extra B vitamins and vitamin D.
- *If you're in your seventies,* get new eyeglasses, and survey your home for loose lamp cords and area rugs. In addition, use a nightlight so that you don't trip in the dark. Fractures, especially hip fractures, are dangerous at this time. Continue taking your supplements. (Courtesy of Cal Orey, "Proper Support," *Energy Times,* April 2001, page 61)

At any age you should pay attention to your bones. Indulge in calcium and your stronger bones will thank you.

What's Your Osteoporosis Risk?

1. Are you Caucasian or Asian? Caucasian and Asian women are most likely to develop osteoporosis, but African-American and Hispanic women are also at significant risk.
2. Have other members of your family suffered osteoporosis or hip fractures? Relatives with this disease indicate you are at risk.
3. Have you broken a bone after age 40? Your bones may be thinning.
4. Have you already experienced menopause? Women can lose up to 20 percent of their bone mass in the five to seven years following menopause, making them more susceptible to osteoporosis.
5. Are you small-framed? Small-boned, thin women are at greater risk. Heavier people have more padding in their hip region, which acts as a cushion that lowers the risk of a fracture.
6. Do you smoke cigarettes? Smoking makes you more prone to bone loss.
7. Are you a couch potato? Inactivity makes your bones grow weaker.
8. Do you take medications that can harm your bones? These include steroids, blood thinners, anticonvulsants, and thyroid medications.
9. Do you imbibe a lot of alcoholic beverages? Drinking too much alcohol interferes with the body's ability to absorb and use bone-boosting calcium and vitamin C.

How You Scored

According to Dr. Ovalle, answering yes to three or more questions indicates moderate risk for osteoporosis. Further evaluation by a health practitioner, including bone density testing, may help evaluate risk.

(Source: National Osteoporosis Foundation)

THE DOC'S SUPPLEMENT LIST

These supplements are what Dr. Ovalle takes to keep her bones healthy and strong.

Supplement	What It Does	Dose
Calcium	This important dietary supplement has been shown to improve bone mass in both men and women	1,500 mg daily
Vitamin D	This vitamin is considered essential for the maintenance of bone health	400 IU for adults daily
Multivitamin-and-mineral supplement	This supplement ensures the adequate intake of other important bone-boosting nutrients	As directed

DR. GABY'S PROPER SUPPORT FOR MEN

ALAN GABY, M.D.

Author of *Preventing and Reversing Osteoporosis* (Prima), Alan Gaby, M.D., is well aware of the fact that bone loss is not just a woman's problem. Men can fall victim to osteoporosis, too.

On a personal level, Dr. Gaby believes exercise is crucial to strong bones. He tries to run 12 miles per week. "It keeps my bones strong. Bone remodels along the lines of stress. If you put physical stress on a bone by pressing on it, then it's forced to get stronger. So running strengthens the bones in the column of the vertebrae and the hips, which are the two main areas where people get fractures," he explains.

Diet-wise, Dr. Gaby lightens up on sugar, caffeine, alcohol, and animal foods, which all can cause bone loss. "Each of them causes loss of calcium through the urine, which means that the bone is breaking down," he says.

He adds, "The conventional wisdom is calcium, estrogen, aerobic exercise, and vitamin D. I realized that there were many, many things that were being completely overlooked even though they were published in research; they were just being forgotten." Dr. Gaby also realizes statistics prove men can be victims of bone loss.

FACTS F.Y.I.

According to the National Institute and Related Bone Diseases—Natural Resource Center:

- One out of eight men over age 50 will have an osteoporosis-related fracture in their lifetime.
- More than 2 million American men suffer from osteoporosis, and millions more are at risk.
- Each year, 80,000 men suffer a hip fracture, and one-third of these men die within a year.

THE DOC'S SUPPLEMENT LIST

So what are some of the other nutrients Dr. Gaby mentions that can help prevent bone loss?

Supplement	What It Does
Vitamin K	Key to bone formation; this vitamin binds calcium to the bone matrix
Boron	This mineral helps metabolism of calcium and magnesium and boosts levels of the bone-building hormones estrogen and testosterone
Manganese	A bone-boosting mineral that aids in maintaining bone cartilage and bone collagen formation

OsteoPrime   Dr. Gaby takes this product, which includes the above nutrients. While it's designed primarily for women, it's good for men, too. "It's a basic multivitamin-and-mineral, but the difference between it and other multivitamins is that it contains four or five nutrients that are very important for bone, either not included in other multiples or not included in adequate amounts," he says.

DR. SIEGEL'S BONE PROTECTION TIPS FOR KIDS

IRWIN M. SIEGEL, M.D. 42

The fact is, exercise is important for kids' bones, muscles, and joints. Getting physical helps children with their weight control, coordination, and balance and builds stronger bones and better-conditioned muscles and other soft tissues that stabilize joints, explains Dr. Irwin M. Siegel, an orthopedic surgeon.

Kids are different from adults. Since they are still growing, there are certain anatomical and physiological differences that make them more injury-prone, explains Dr. Siegel. "They suffer more soft tissue injuries despite the fact that their ligaments are often stronger than their bones." However, they do recover faster than adults. Here are some common injuries and important bone protection strategies you can put to use.

Sprains and Strains. It's common to strain or sprain the ligaments or other soft tissues around the joint without having a severe enough injury to break a bone. The thing that you have to be careful about with children is that you don't overlook an unrecognized cartilage injury. (This is not apparent on an X-ray.)

Smart Strategy. "You always look for more than a sprain or strain. That's diagnosis by exclusion." In other words, doctors like Dr. Siegel will try to rule out an underlying cartilage problem, which can cause a growth deformity at the site of the injury.

Overuse Injuries. Kids can develop swimmer's shoulder (where there is irritation of the shoulder tendon) or jumper's knee (where there is an irritation of the tendon that attaches to the kneecap that attaches the tibia bone to the lower leg). Also, they get Little League elbow (which is caused by repetitive active throwing, particularly in pitchers, which causes stress to the elbow). Children whose bony structures are immature are vulnerable to chipping bone. And they can even have loose cartilage in their joints.

Smart Strategy. "Limit the amount of time a Little Leaguer pitches. You've got to protect the elbow. No more than five or six innings should be pitched each week, and at least four or five days off should be allowed between games," suggests Dr. Siegel.

Tennis Elbow. Tennis elbow is common in both children and adults. It's an irritation of the elbow due to a defective backhand. But common sense comes to the rescue, according to Dr. Siegel.

Smart Strategies. Tennis elbow is remedied by improving the backhand stroke, using a double-handed backhand stroke; and taking some lessons so you play your backhand with your elbow and wrist rigid. Also, using a large racket made of a springy material designed to absorb stress and using a tennis elbow strap and forearm-strengthening exercises such as wrist curls can help stave off recurrences.

Knee Injuries. Another problem, especially in teenage girls, is irritation of the cartilage of the kneecap. It's so common that it has been referred to as runner's knee. Often it happens because girls are knock-kneed, which causes unusual wear on the femur. Sometimes, the first sign of pain is felt after crossing the knees.

Smart Strategies. Rest and ice are recommended. Vitamin C and anti-inflammatory drugs such as aspirin can be helpful. Occasionally a knee brace may be beneficial.

Slipped Hip. This is an injury (most common in athletic boys and in running or contact sports) where the ball part of the hip slips off the shaft at the growth zone. It is about 50 percent bilateral—happening on both sides.

Smart Strategy. It is a disabling injury if not recognized early with an X-ray and treated vigorously.

THE DOC'S SUPPLEMENT LIST

These nutrients are what Dr. Siegel recommends to help kids heal faster if they get an injury.

Supplement	What It Does
Vitamin C	This antioxidant vitamin helps heal the soft tissues and acts as an anti-inflammatory agent
Vitamin E	Works as an antioxidant vitamin that decreases inflammation

Safety Smarts: Vitamin C: If you take too much, it can cause gastrointestinal problems.

Doc's Rx for Healing Yourself

- Take calcium and vitamin D supplements to improve bone mass in both men and women.
- Consider soy supplements and foods before, during, and after menopause to maintain your bones.
- Limit sweets, refined foods, salt, alcohol, and caffeine, all of which can cause bone loss.

- Get a bone density test at 50—or earlier if you are at high risk for osteoporosis.
- If you are at high risk for osteoporosis, consult with your doctor for preventive drug therapy options and participate in a regular exercise program, such as walking or lifting light weights, to strengthen your muscles, bones, and joints.
- Take vitamin K, which is key to bone formation.
- Opt for the bone-boosting minerals boron and manganese.
- Beware of kids' common injuries and if a child gets a sports injury, don't hesitate to consult your doctor as a preventive measure.
- If a child has a minor injury, use the RICE method (rest, ice, compression wrap, and elevation) and vitamin C to reduce swelling and shorten time of recovery.

BIOS

Alan Gaby, M.D., professor of nutrition at Bastyr University. At 51, he resides in Seattle, Washington. He is the author of several books including *The Book of Natural Healing* (Prima). Also, he is a formulator of OsteoPrime, a bone formula sold in health food stores.

Melba Iris Ovalle, M.D., is a board-certified rheumatologist and medical director of Evanston Northwestern Healthcare Osteoporosis Center in Highland Park, Illinois. She graduated from Boston University Medical School and did her medical residency and fellowship training in rheumatology at Albert Einstein/Montefiore Medical Center in New York. She lives in Deerfield, Illinois, with her husband and three daughters and three dachshunds. Additional information on Dr. Ovalle and the Osteoporosis Center as well as valuable links can be found at her web site: www.doctorovalle.com.

Irwin M. Siegel, M.D., is an orthopedic surgeon and an associate professor in the departments of neurology, orthopedics, and physical medicine and rehabilitation at Rush–Presbyterian–St. Luke's Medical Center in Chicago, Illinois. Dr. Siegel graduated from Northwestern University College of Medicine. He is also the author of *All About Muscle, All About Bone,* and *All About Joints* (all published by Demos Medical Publishers). He resides in Chicago, Illinois, is 74, is married, and has four children and twenty-four grandchildren.

PART V

All in the Head

Five years ago, I woke up at dawn in Kauai, Hawaii. I sauntered into the kitchen to join my host in a cup of java. After that I strolled out to her backyard. I sat by the pool amid several laid-back cats basking in the warm sun. After I took a dip in the water, I set out to an isolated beach where I sat cross-legged on the sand and gazed out at the ocean's waves. I was cool, calm, and on another planet.

According to the doctors in Part V, "All in the Head," you'll be able to find this type of nirvana without going to the Hawaiian Islands. If you would like a way to handle your stress and anxiety, you'll find out how to calm your frazzled nerves on the following pages.

Question: What do anxiety, brain wellness, depression, headaches, insomnia, and stress have in common? Answer: They are all linked by the nervous system, which is the central processing unit of the body. And you can think yourself well by doing as these doctors do.

Dr. Harold Bloomfield, author of *Healing Anxiety Naturally* (Harper Trade), declares: "The purpose of life is the expansion of happiness." And by following his anti-anxiety strategies you will be able to join him on the road to inner peace.

Drs. Jay Lombard and Russell Blaylock provide brain-boosting diet, supplement, and lifestyle strategies to keep your brain working at its optimal best as you age.

On the East Coast, Norman Rosenthal, M.D., will explain how he fought and won the battle against the winter blues.

Drs. Seymour Diamond, M.D., and Alexander Mauskop, M.D., help people every day to prevent and treat headaches. And with Dr. Lauren Broch's practical remedies for getting adequate z's, you should sleep like a baby.

Medical experts such as William F. Fry, M.D., and Joan Borysenko, Ph.D., and psychologists John Amodeo, Jane Greer, and Stanley Coren will show you that humor, taking time-out, love, patience, and pets are the kinds of things that have healing power. And all of these doctors provide healthful ways that can help soothe your nerves!

18

Anxiety

Q AND A WITH DR. BLOOMFIELD

HAROLD BLOOMFIELD, M.D.

When Dr. Harold Bloomfield was completing medical school he had an unforgettable wake-up call. During a bout of Zen-like soul-searching about whether or not he wanted to be a doctor, he sought professional guidance.

One doctor's visit later, he was labeled "anxious" and "depressed." When Bloomfield told the doctor he was thinking of traveling to India to study meditation, the psychiatrist said it was only a quick fix. "I need to put you on antidepressants and Valium," the psychiatrist said. Bloomfield sought a second opinion. This doctor told him he needed psychoanalysis. When Bloomfield saw a third shrink, a Jungian analyst, he heard positive feedback regarding his dream to go to India.

As a result, Dr. Bloomfield went to India and taught meditation. One year later he became a psychiatrist. (Today he sees patients, many of them high-profile, about 20 hours per week.) His past personal awakening has made him a more down-to-earth doctor who can relate to other people who need to learn how to cope with stress, anxiety, and depression.

In an enjoyable chat with the well-grounded and spiritual Dr. Bloomfield, author of *Natural Healing for Anxiety and Depression* (Hay House), I asked him a variety of questions about anxiety. The answers he gave not only were candid and heartfelt, they can be solutions for plenty of people like you and me, and even for busy doctors.

Q. *Do you see a lot of doctors who are stressed out or anxious?*
A. It's unbelievable. That's like an oxymoron. Yes, yes, yes. The average general practitioner now in an HMO setting has five minutes per patient. They have that pressure of practicing poor medicine. In this generation there is a loss of self-esteem for physicians. They are less esteemed by society.

Q. *Why? Because we're taking so much control in our own hands and going for a second opinion as you did?*
A. Exactly, which is good. It is important for each of us to be more responsible for our own health, ask a lot of questions, and be our own advocate. And the doctors are not patronizing and authoritarian; they take time to be not only thorough in their evaluation but thorough in their discussion with the patient about their diagnosis and potential range of treatments—especially when it comes to anxiety.

Q. *What is your number-one calming advice to chill out?*
A. If I had only one, and assuming people would follow through on it, I would have people take the Transcendental Meditation (TM) program (a form of meditation, based on Hindu philosophy, that uses a mantra that you repeat silently as you meditate). It's been shown in research to be quite unique in that it evokes a deep state of rest, twice as deep as the deepest point of a night's sleep, while the mind remains alert within.

And that state of restful alertness is the exact opposite of the stress and anxiety that we see in our culture where people are tense and tired. Rather than eliciting a fight-or-flight response, it elicits a stay-and-play response.

Q. *Do you practice TM yourself?*
A. I do TM twice daily. I used to be a very uptight, anxious person.

Q. *When you were finishing up medical school and saw a Jungian analyst who told you that your idea to practice meditation in India would be a good experience, why was that a "nervous breakthrough" for you?*
A. Because I had grown up to be the family hero. To be compliant. I had fulfilled those wishes of German-Jewish refugees from the Nazi holocaust—their dreams for their son. Then I realized, however, that I was not a happy camper. I was really stressed out. I also saw that there was an alternative. People who practiced TM twice daily over time become less and less vulnerable to stress. I wanted to experience that myself and then teach it to my patients.

Q. *Why do you advise your patients to try meditation, exercise, dietary changes, and so on, to calm anxiety?*
A. Because we know that those factors are the number-one risk factors in whether we remain healthy and blissful, or sickly and stressful.

Q. *Isn't it easier to pop a Valium to chill out?*
A. Oh, sure. In terms of the immediate response, pop a Valium and you're going to feel calm. The problem is, all the benzodiazepines within two days develop dependency. And you can have rebound anxiety. After a while they create their own need. You have millions of people who are legally getting these drugs from their physicians. They are highly addicted.

Q. *Psychologically and physically?*
A. Absolutely. The problem is, we use benzodiazepines as tranquilizers in the day as well as sleeping pills at night. What happens is that people start to lose faith in their own healing capacity. They think of themselves more and more as "I've got to have that Valium" or "I've got to have that sleeping pill or I won't get to sleep." The rebound insomnia, the rebound anxiety.

So I've been looking for alternatives ever since my days at Yale. What are the alternatives that we can offer people who are suffering from mild to moderate anxiety (which is 99 percent of us), as opposed to the ones that show up in the emergency room with panic attacks or have a more serious mental illness going on? To use the benzodiazepines is like using an elephant gun to swat a fly.

Q. *Yes, but for people who have high-stress jobs (from doctors to journalists) it seems easier to turn to Valium and just get on with it.*
A. It works. I'm not so much passing a value judgment as I am wanting people to know the pluses and minuses of any choice they make. For example, whatever benzodiazepines you're taking, over time you'll need more and more for the same effect.

Q. *Other than TM, how do you stay calm, especially with your busy schedule?*
A. Ever since my books on herbal medicine I've become a world-wide herb hunter. I recently got back from India where I was studying the herbs used in Ayurveda medicine [an Indian method of disease prevention achieved through balance].

The next big herbal superstar is a synergistic formula of nine herbs. It is being researched right now at the University of California at San Diego School of Medicine. The results are showing that it is a fantastic treatment for generalized anxiety disorder (GAD). It is not addictive and has no side effects.

Q. *So what three anti-anxiety herbs should I take so I can be a stress-free journalist?*
A. It would be a combination of three things. Indian valerian has a calming sedative quality to it. If you have the right amount it's not going to make you sleepy; it will help calm you down. Then I would take ashwaganda, which is what's called an adaptogen; if you take it over time, deadlines will be less stressful. Your amygdala (that emotional center of our brain) will start to calm down. A lot of us develop hyperactive amygdalas; we're just buzzed all the time. The third herb, called brahmi, works to have our nat-

ural levels of GABA (a neurochemical in our brain) restored in the brain, which helps you think more calmly.

Q. *Several of your books are about finding inner peace in general. How can that help you to chill out?*
A. Every one at a certain point in their life, especially in Western culture, really develops almost a craving to be at peace amidst all the nonstop, future-shock, 24/7 overload. *Quintessential peace* is the term I use, and it refers to peace in all five sectors of our self: in our body, relationships, emotions, intellect, and spirituality. All five are important aspects to be paid attention to.

Q. *What are your most helpful strategies for cultivating inner peace?*
A. Learn TM because it will make a great difference in your life. I would put you on Worry Free™ [a combination of herbs to help balance the mind and the emotions] for at least a six-month period to help your brain replenish itself. Number three, I would have people doing deep breathing exercises. Move into peace, whether it's going through a walk in the park or on the Stairmaster. Changing your physiology changes your psychology. Or your can train yourself not to be in the past but to be in the here and now.

Q. *Will all these things help me and other people to shut off their brain or "cut off their head"?*
A. Absolutely. I was about to cut off my head before I learned TM because my mind would not quit. And I have one of these minds that if it wasn't for those 20 minutes twice a day where it unplugs I would be a basket case.

DOCTOR'S LINGO

Stress response: A physical response triggered by the sensitivity of our sympathetic system, which jump-starts the fight-or-flight reaction. When the pressure is on, our pulse rate, respiration, muscle tension, and blood pressure can soar. When huge waves of anxiety hit, clinical anxiety disorders—including panic attacks and phobias—can happen.

THE DOC'S SUPPLEMENT LIST

For mild to moderate anxiety, Dr. Bloomfield recommends herbal remedies combined with good anti-anxiety habits. These "deserve to be considered before synthetic drugs because of their relative safety and fewer side effects," he says.

Supplement	What It Does
Brahmi	An Ayurvedic herb to help relieve anxiety
Ginseng/ Ashwaganda	These herbs can help to strengthen the nervous system and protect against stress
Kava	This nutrient can relieve mild to moderate anxiety as effectively as Valium-like tranquilizers but without sedation, memory impairment, or addiction
Skullcap	This herb is an antispasmodic that eases muscular pain from stress
St. John's wort	Extracts of hypericum can be just as effective as antidepressants, which are for mild to moderate depression, and can also be used to rid one of anxiety
Valerian	Valerian root can provide a good night's sleep without morning hangover or the rebound insomnia of prescription sleeping pills

Safety Smarts: Kava: Do not take it if you are taking benzodiazepines or mix kava with alcohol. St. John's wort: It may cause sun sensitiviy. Do not mix with other antidepressants. Valerian: Do not take if you're using other sleep- or mood-enhancing medications.

BREATHING RIGHT WITH DR. REECE

THOMAS REECE, N.D., D.O.

44

Ever notice that when you are anxious people will tell you to take deep breaths? Well, Dr. Thomas Reece will tell you that he does just that for a whopping twenty-four minutes a day!

He turns to a Traditional Chinese Medicine "Qi Gong" exercise that utilizes visualization, movement, meditation, and breath regulation to promote Qi flow throughout the body. (Qi is the vital life energy of the body. Qi flows through energy pathways called meridians. Charts on acupuncture show these meridian pathways.)

This exercise cleanses the body and improves and balances the nervous system. "Performing Qi Gong induces alpha brain waves and thus decreases the fight, flight, and fright response of the sympathetic nervous system. This makes Qi Gong a good anti-anxiety exercise," he says.

"You can do the exercise for a shorter time period. Even four breaths would be beneficial. It is said that it takes performing the exercise for 30 days straight to become proficient at it. You will realize it when you achieve a good breath," explains Dr. Reece.

Here, Dr. Reece's step-by-step personal breathing exercise, called the Diamond Palm Breathing Exercise, which can help you, too, to relax day by day.

1. Stand with arms at your sides.
2. Inhale as much as you can while making fists with your hands.
3. Hold breath at top of sternum such that there is no tension on your throat. Hold as long as possible.
4. Release breath and open hands simultaneously. Keep lips relaxed so exhaled air creates the sound horses or lions make when chuffing.

   Perform this exercise for 24 minutes a day, one arm's length from a tree or inside wall. Stop if you become light-headed.

CALM DOWN WITH DR. AMODEO

JOHN AMODEO, PH.D.

As contributing editor of *Complete Woman* magazine, I have often turned to psychotherapist Dr. John Amodeo for his words of wisdom. Each time the doctor is centered, which certainly must help when he listens to his patients' relationship problems. According to Amodeo, these four strategies help him to chill:

- *Massage.* "It's especially helpful when I've been writing a lot," says Dr. Amodeo. "My neck and shoulders can get tense sitting in front of the computer screen for hours at a time. Not all massages are alike. I'm fortunate to see someone who applies just the right amount of pressure for my body."
- *Yoga.* Dr. Amodeo feels that "a little yoga every morning helps ease me into my day without caffeine. It's relaxing and tunes up my energy as well. A longer class is helpful if I'm especially stressed. It provides a wonderful combination of tranquillity and energy."
- *Working out at the gym.* "If I'm writing a good part of the day, I find it essential to work out on the fitness machines. This reminds me that I have a body!" says Dr. Amodeo. "Writing is very sedentary and although I feel enlivened being in the creative process, it can sometimes be tiring. Working out gives me energy for the remainder of the day."
- *Walking in nature.* Dr. Amodeo finds it "very rejuvenating to walk around the lake, go to the ocean, or visit the redwood forest. Walking through nature is an enriching meditation for me. Letting in beauty fills my soul and eases whatever worries or anxieties may be bouncing around inside me."

RESEARCH IN A NUTSHELL

One doctor has recognized that there are healing powers of nature. A study from Emory University in Atlanta, Georgia, suggests that there is a link between health and environment. Studies have shown that landscapes, plants, pets, and wilderness experiences may have health benefits beyond exercising. More research is needed to pinpoint which kinds of nature contact are most healthful. (Frumkin, F., "Beyond toxicity: human health and the natural environment." *American Journal of Preventive Medicine.* 2001; 20 (3):234–240)

DOC'S RX TO HEAL YOURSELF

- Practice Transcendental Meditation.
- Opt for anti-anxiety herbs such as brahmi, kava, Saint John's wort, and valerian.
- Do breathing exercises regularly.
- Chill out by using anti-anxiety techniques daily: yoga, massage, workouts, or tuning in to nature.

BIOS

John Amodeo, Ph.D., is a psychotherapist in private practice in the San Francisco Bay Area. He received his Ph.D. from the Institute of Transpersonal Psychology in Palo Alto, California. He is the author of *The Authentic Heart: An Eightfold Path to Midlife Love* (John Wiley & Sons) and *Love and Betrayal* (Ballantine). Dr. Amodeo has more than twenty years' experience assisting individuals and couples with their journey toward satisfying relationships. At 51, he lives in Sebastopol, California.

Harold Bloomfield, M.D., is a 56-year-old Yale-trained psychiatrist, author of more than fifteen books, such as *How to Survive the Loss of a Love* (Prelude Press), *Making Peace with Your Past* (Harper Trade), and his latest book, *Making Peace with God* (Putnam), coauthored with Philip Goldberg, Ph.D. He works and resides in Del Mar, California, is married, and has three children.

Thomas Reece, N.D., D.O., is board certified in osteopathic family practice medicine. He received his doctorate in naturopathic medicine from the National College of Naturopathic Medicine and his doctorate in osteopathic medicine from Kirksville College of Osteopathic Medicine. He has a current practice in Scottsdale, Arizona.

19

Brain Wellness

DR. LOMBARD'S ULTIMATE PLAN

JAY LOMBARD, D.O.

Dr. Jay Lombard, a neurologist and author of the *Brain Wellness Plan* (Kensington), knows too well that most neurological diseases are progressive. That means the majority of patients he sees, 99 percent, have neurological or psychiatric conditions such as Alzheimer's, Parkinson's, or depression.

His interest in brain wellness stems from his father, who died from a stroke. "It was the initial event that got me interested in neurology. Here was a man that was previously articulate and intelligent, and he wasn't able to speak after his stroke. A stroke is a brain injury event," he explains. That gave Dr. Lombard the desire to see if he could help other people who suffer from neurological problems.

The patients whom he sees are of all ages. He sees children with autism to attention deficit disorder and adults with the following disorders:

- *Alzheimer's disease.* A brain disease that affects proper brain function. Symptoms include memory loss and confusion.

- *Parkinson's disease.* A brain disease that destroys the brain cells that affect an individual's ability to move. Symptoms include slowness of movement and trembling.
- *Depression.* A brain disorder that includes major or clinical depression and manic-depressive illness. Symptoms include feelings of sadness, crying, fatigue, hopelessness, and thoughts of suicide.
- *Dementia.* A brain disorder or disease that causes deterioration of the mind. Symptoms include memory loss to insanity.

SMART PREVENTIVE STRATEGIES

According to Dr. Lombard, here's how he personally practices brain wellness.

- *Destress.* "I destress by having a sense of purpose in my life: healing people. I have very strong relationships with my friends, family, and wife that are supportive. I do light weight training and aerobics. The main thing it does is reduce cortisol."
- *Consume fish oils.* In addition, Dr. Lombard believes that a diet high in essential fatty acids is brain food. "Because the major composition of the brain is fat. And different fats affect the membranes of the brain. So the more polyunsaturated fats in a diet, the better the cell membranes function in the brain." He eats fish three or four times a week.
- *Consume more colorful vegetables.* "The color of vegetables is very important. The more colorful the vegetables are, the more [antioxidant rich] polyphenols you will get. [Antioxidants] will get rid of the [damaging] free radical scavengers, which is helpful for brain health and general health," explains Dr. Lombard.
- *Use it or lose it.* "The brain needs exercise. My life is very stimulating," says Dr. Lombard.

Anti-Aging Antics of Dr. Blaylock

RUSSELL L. BLAYLOCK, M.D.

Dr. Russell Blaylock has a special interest in Parkinson's disease. Why? The frightening disease hit home. "My father died of Parkinson's disease. My mother is in her eighties now, and she has Parkinson's," he says.

"We're beginning to see these neurodegenerative diseases in married couples. There is some concern because they are living in the same household and they either are exposed to the same environmental toxic elements, eat the same diet, or share some infectious disease," explains Dr. Blaylock, who has been interested in brain function for his entire career.

Dr. Blaylock has a nutritional practice and specializes in neurodegenerative diseases such as Parkinson's and Alzheimer's. People come to Dr. Blaylock for prevention if their parents or some family member had one of these diseases.

"Nutritional treatments equal anything that the pharmaceutical companies have. Plus, it's a lot fewer side effects and complications," he points out. "When you look at the cause of Alzheimer's and Parkinson's they all have shared characteristics. So what we try to do is change that.

"There is a high free radical damage [free radicals are unstable molecules that result from your body's metabolic processes, and also derive from buildup in toxins from the environment] to the brain that produces these disorders," says Dr. Blaylock, who believes supplements may help slow the course of the neurodegenerative disorder or even prevent the onset.

THE DOC'S SUPPLEMENT LIST

Here's some nutrients Dr. Blaylock uses himself to prevent developing Parkinson's disease.

Supplement	What It Does
Alpha-lipoic acid	An antioxidant that prevents free radical damage, increases brain cell energy production
CoQ_{10}	Can bypass energy deficits and prevent damage by certain toxins (inflammatory chemicals in the brain), thanks to its antioxidant action
Vitamin C	Like vitamin E, this antioxidant fights free radical damage in brain cells
Vitamin E	This antioxidant vitamin fights free radical damage in brain cells
L-carnitine	An amino acid that can bypass energy deficits and prevent damage by certain toxins
Glutathione	An antioxidant that increases the ability of cells to build energy. In Parkinson's this antioxidant falls dramatically low, and as it's lowered, the free radicals start destroying cells

Safety Smarts: Alpha-lipoic acid: If you are diabetic and taking insulin, lipoic acid can lower your blood glucose level, which may lower your need for medications. Talk to your doctor. Vitamin C: If you take too much, it can cause gastrointestinal problems.

DR. LOFTUS'S MEMORY TECHNIQUES

ELIZABETH LOFTUS, PH.D.

Ever see the unforgettable *Seinfeld* episode in which the characters become distraught because they can't remember where they parked their car in the parking lot? Well, cognitive psychologist Elizabeth Loftus, Ph.D., exercises her brain with these three easy memory techniques that can help you to keep your memory sharp and may even prevent a missing car mishap.

- *Repeat. Repeat.* One way to maximize memory is to learn how to rehearse what you've just seen. If you don't want to forget that you parked your car on Floor 6, Row B, try this technique, recommends Dr. Loftus. "You can get out of the car and say aloud to yourself, "6B, 6B, 6B." Wait five minutes, and say 6B again. Then wait five more minutes and say 6B again. That is called "spaced practice." The best method is the "expanding rehearsal pattern." "Say 6B aloud to yourself, 6B; wait a minute, say 6B again; wait ten minutes. . . . Each interval gets longer and longer. That expanding pattern of rehearsal leads to the best recall," insists Dr. Loftus. The key is to say it aloud to yourself often.
- *Create an image.* Another basic tool for improving memory is the use of imagery. Creating vivid images can help you to remember. "If you park your car in space 4D, turn the letter into a word such as *door*. That will help you remember where you parked," explains Dr. Loftus.
- *Leave cues.* Or you can try leaving "retrieval cues" to help jog your memory. Says Dr. Loftus, "Sometimes I leave a stool in front of the door when I'm about to leave home. I remember that the stool is there to cue a memory (for example, 'Don't forget to leave a check for the housekeeper'). Retrieval cues will help jog your memory."

DOCS' RX TO HEAL YOURSELF

- Destress to lower damaging effects of the hormone cortisol.
- Include fish oils by either eating fish or taking supplements for better cell membrane function in your brain.
- Eat antioxidant-rich vegetables to get rid of damaging free radicals.
- Exercise your brain with stimulation.
- Opt for antioxidant supplements—alpha-lipoic acid, CoQ_{10}, vitamins C and E, L-carnitine, and glutathione—to help prevent free radical damage, increase brain cell energy, and stave off degenerative neurodiseases.
- Use memory exercises to stimulate your mind.

BIOS

Russell L. Blaylock, M.D., is a board-certified neurosurgeon who completed his medical training at the Louisiana State University School of Medicine in New Orleans, Louisiana. Dr. Blaylock, at 55, has a clinic called Advanced Nutritional Concepts in Flowood, Mississippi. He is also the author of *Excitotoxins* (Health Press). He resides in Richland, Mississippi, with his wife and their two children.

Elizabeth Loftus, Ph.D., is a cognitive psychologist in the psychology department at the University of Washington in Seattle. The over-50 doctor currently resides in Washington. She is the author of *Eyewitness Testimony* (Harvard University Press). Web site: http://faculty.washington.edu/eloftus.

Jay Lombard, D.O., is a 40-year-old director of the Brain Behavior Center in Rockland County, New York. He is the author of *Brain Wellness Plan* (Kensington) and assistant clinical professor at Cornell Medical School. Web site: www.braincures.com.

20

Seasonal Affective Disorder

BEATING THE WINTER BLUES WITH DR. ROSENTHAL

NORMAN ROSENTHAL, M.D.

Back in the mid-1970s, Dr. Norman Rosenthal relished the long dog-day afternoons in New York City during the summer. "I had boundless energy. Then daylight savings time came. All of a sudden it was dark in the afternoon. I remember feeling a sense of dread. And then winter set in. My energy level declined. But I persevered through the winter," he recalls. Strangely, when spring came and the days got longer, his energy returned and his gloom-and-doom attitude disappeared.

Dr. Rosenthal was suffering from seasonal affective disorder (SAD), a condition (which the doctor coined) that causes low moods and energy, especially in the winter months. And, experts largely agree, the farther you are from the equator, the more common SAD—or its milder form, the "winter blues"—is.

How did Dr. Rosenthal and about 15 to 25 million Americans get this disorder? Researchers link SAD to melatonin, a sleep-related hormone that the tiny pineal gland (located at the base of the brain) produces and releases in the evening or at times of diminished light, according to the National Mental Health Association (NMHA) in Alexandria, Virginia. Its secretion peaks in the middle of the night, when we experience our heaviest sleep; evidently, production of the hormone is also particularly high during winter's shortened daylight hours.

Winter depression often begins in early adulthood, and four times as many women as men are affected. In fact, for most SAD sufferers, January and February are the cruelest months.

If you are SAD-prone, turn this season into a time of positive self-help. Dr. Rosenthal can help you see the light.

LIGHTEN UP

One important treatment is to expose people to more light. The way to do it, explains Dr. Rosenthal, is to use a light box because you pack a lot of light into a small amount of space. Therefore, people get a lot of light all at once, which is what these people seem to need.

"The first studies, which took place in the early 1980s, were extremely exciting, because one by one, we saw these patients respond to the bright light treatment even within a couple of days. Their symptoms would reverse and they would become more energetic, they wouldn't have such a ravenous appetite, and their weight would go down," says Dr. Rosenthal.

"Around that time when I began to experiment with my patients, I began to experiment with myself. In my bedroom I had a big light box that I would turn on early in the morning, and I personally experienced the mood lift as a result of the light exposure," he adds.

The intensity of light used in the therapy is important. Current therapy uses 10,000-lux white fluorescent light, with ultraviolet (UV) filters, usually mounted in a box. Dr. Rosenthal's patients begin with 15-minute exposures and work up to a maximum of 45 minutes, ideally in the morning, though many patients use the light box twice a day. (Dr. Rosenthal varies the intensity of light based upon many factors such as time of year, the weather, and how he is feeling.)

In addition to light box treatment, Dr. Rosenthal uses a dawn simulator, a lamp or overhead light set to gradually increase in intensity from 4:30 to 6 A.M. "It turns on the lamp gradually on a winter morning to simulate the effect of the shade on your bedroom window on a summer day," adds Dr. Rosenthal.

"In that way for the last many years I have functioned very adequately through the winter. I also plan vacations in the South, and I take them in the winter rather than the summer—that's when I need them the most," he says.

Dr. Rosenthal also exercises regularly with a personal trainer. Outdoor exercise provides you with increased natural daylight; exercise can help you lose weight, and after exercise the body feels relaxed yet not tired.

"Meanwhile, it turns out that my wife also has SAD, and she has used the light every winter. And one day when my son was in high school he came to me and said, 'You know, I think I'm seasonal, too. I'm dozing off at my homework, I'm going for junk food.' I thought for sure he was just copying his parents." But the winter blues were indeed affecting Dr. Rosenthal's son as well.

"Thanks to the light box he got through college with no difficulty. And, once again, thanks to his regular treatment of his winter difficulties he was able to get through medical school," says Dr. Rosenthal.

It turns out that the doctor's son is hardly alone. Many young people suffer from this problem, according to Dr. Rosenthal. "We estimate that one million middle and high school children suffer from SAD. College freshman suffer tremendously because their parents are no longer getting them up and going in the early morning, so they're missing out on the morning light. And they're probably becoming depressed. So I have greatly improved my own life and that of my wife and son."

CHANGE YOUR ENVIRONMENT

While most people with mild winter doldrums do not need light therapy, changing your environment can lift your mood. Dr.

Rosenthal suggests enhancing light levels at home or in the workplace by installing more lights on the ceiling or placing more lamps in the room.

Additionally, winter vacations and relocating to a sunnier climate, reports Dr. Rosenthal, are some more dramatic solutions that several of his patients have chosen. For other patients, simply warming up helps, too. Warmth strategies to try? Turn up the thermostat, use electric blankets, drink warm beverages, and layer clothing.

I can personally attest that these tips work well. Since I have moved to a location where the winters are cold, it's a good feeling to make a fire, crank up the waterbed heater, layer my clothing in all-natural fabrics, and sip herbal tea.

And sometimes, ancient remedies are best. According to Rosenthal, the Roman physician A. Cornelius Celsus gave the following advice to melancholics during the reign of Emperor Tiberius: Live in rooms full of light; indulge in cheerful conversation and amusements; listen to music.

FACT F.Y.I.

According to the National Mental Health Association:

• More than 17 million Americans experience depression in one form or another every year.

DOC'S RX TO HEAL YOURSELF

• If you have SAD, opt for light therapy.
• Exercise will make you feel better.
• Enhance light levels at home and in the workplace.
• Opt for winter vacations.
• Live in rooms full of light and amusement.

Bio

Norman Rosenthal, M.D., is a clinical professor of psychiatry at Georgetown University. He did his medical training in South Africa and currently has a private practice in Rockville, Maryland. He is the author of *Winter Blues* (Guilford Publications) and *The Emotional Revolution* (Citadel Press). He resides in Bethesda, Maryland. At 50, he is married and has one son.Web site: www.normanrosenthal.com.

21

Headaches

Q & A WITH DR. DIAMOND

SEYMOUR DIAMOND, M.D.

Several years ago, I wrote an article on how to prevent holiday headaches for a national health magazine. I interviewed Dr. Seymour Diamond, a renowned headache expert. It was as though I had called a dial-a-wizard on headache prevention and treatment. Recently, I spoke with the doctor who knows headaches.

Q. *Why the big interest in headaches?*
A. I became a doctor and the headache interest developed later. In the 1960s I did some work with chronic daily headache and chronic pain with the antidepressant drugs. I found that patients got relief. It helped to cut down and prevent their headaches. Nobody really noted this before. In fact, I say in many of my lectures, "If these drugs were discovered today and we didn't know they were antidepressants they would be called analgesics." In other words, they have an analgesic property without being a narcotic or sedative. And I became extremely interested from that point of view.

Q. *What type of headache do you see most often?*
A. We see migraine, clusters, and chronic daily headaches.

Q. *You once told me that 90 percent of all headaches are tension-related. But I recently read that all of these types of headaches can be combined. Can you have all three?*
A. Yes, that's what I'm calling the chronic daily headaches. But clusters are not usually combined except rarely.

Q. *So how does your procedure for headache treatment work?*
A. I sit down and spend an hour with you. I want to know how many kinds of headaches you have. I want to know where it's located, because if it's migraine it's usually a one-sided headache or if it's clusters it's usually around the eye. If it's a tension headache it's all over the head. I want to know how often you get it.

Q. *What about a killer headache right above the eyes in the center of the forehead—where I get them?*
A. That's probably a tension type of headache. How often do you get it?

Q. *Whenever I'm stressed out. What type of headache is that?*
A. It's probably a tension type of headache. [He laughs.] I would want to know how long the headache lasts. Clusters last 1 to 3 hours while migraines usually last 8 to 24 hours. Tension headaches can be variable.

Q. *After a consultation you get a handle on what type of headache it is, right?*
A. It fits a pattern after a while.

Q. *So the majority of headaches probably fit into one of the three categories: tension, cluster, or migraine?*
A. Yes. I love to see difficult cases.

SUCCESS STORY

Dr. Diamond treated a 32-year-old married prominent contemporary artist who suffered from daily headaches.

"She started off with migraines, which were intermittent. They occurred on the right side of her head. She had nausea and vomiting. She was getting them about three or four times a month. Then they became more frequent. She also developed what we call a daily headache in a different character than the migraine headache. It was what we call a chronic tension headache.

"When she finally saw me she was completely incapacitated by her headache problem. She couldn't work because she had a constant daily headache. She was taking excessive amounts of over-the-counter medicines. She was prescribed an excessive amount of pain relievers by the physician who was treating her. Many doctors treat the pain and not the source of the headache.

"There's no way any medicines I would give her would be successful without my first hospitalizing her and comfortably getting her off the pain relievers. She would have withdrawal. Once we got her off the drugs that were causing part of the problem, her headaches did get better, but she was still getting headaches that needed further therapy. We used a combination of an antidepressant for her daily headaches [tricyclic antidepressant] along with a beta blocker [which stabilizes the blood vessels] to help her migraine headaches. It's interesting that once we got her off the daily narcotics and caffeine-containing drugs, she was able to distinguish when she was getting a migraine. We were able to give her one of these new triptan drugs (a new class of anti-migraine prescription drugs such as sumatriptan, brand name Imitrix, that block migraine) to take when she got a migraine attack. Actually, they're like miracle drugs. They reverse the migraine. [These drugs can cause problems if you have high blood pressure or heart disease. Be sure to discuss side effects with your doctor.]

"Then we did some nondrug methods: cognitive therapy—going into psychological reasons why she might be having stress and other factors influencing her headache. We used some biofeedback, where we use machines to illustrate to the person what is happening. Then we use certain self-hypnotic exercises to train them how to control it. The outcome: This woman is back painting. She's selling her paintings for hundreds of thousands of dollars. At this point, the only thing she is on is the beta blocker and triptam drugs."

Translation: If you, like Dr. Diamond's patients, suffer migraines, take heart—you're not alone.

Facts F.Y.I.

According to the National Headache Foundation:

- If both your parents had migraines, you have a 75 percent chance of suffering them.
- If only one of your parents is a migraine sufferer, your migraine risk is still 50 percent.
- If only a distant relative has migraines, your risk sinks to 20 percent.
- About 70 percent of all migraine sufferers are women.
- Roughly 60 percent of women's migraines are linked to their menstrual cycle. Attacks may occur several days before, during, or immediately after menses.

Second Opinion: Supplemental Strategies with Dr. Mauskop

ALEXANDER MAUSKOP, M.D.

While effective triptan drug therapy has revolutionized treatment for migraines, some people, perhaps even you, may be wary of potential side effects (from raising blood pressure or causing dizziness). That's why in Dr. Alexander Mauskop's practice he uses many alternative methods such as herbal and mineral remedies and acupuncture.

"When patients come to see me, I give them a list of options of treatments, starting with nondrug approaches ending with drugs, which I use a lot, too," explains Dr. Mauskop. "This is a menu.

The more of these things you pick, the better you are going to feel," he says.

Included in Dr. Mauskop's headache prevention menu are the following:

- *Aerobic exercise.* How can aerobics affect migraines? "One, it relieves the effects of stress. Two, it may release some endorphin in your brain—so-called runner's high, which is also a natural painkiller substance that your brain generates. And the third mechanism is that it has been shown to improve circulation of blood in your brain. Migraines are often caused by prolonged constriction of the blood vessels, and then it leads to a migraine when the blood vessels dilate, throb, and hurt. So if you improve circulation in your brain, your blood vessels are much more flexible," explains Dr. Mauskop. "Many patients will tell me, 'If I exercise I get fewer headaches.' And an occasional one will say, 'As soon as the headache starts coming on I go for a jog and the headache goes away.' Although in some migraine patients a headache can get worse during an attack."
- *Biofeedback.* Like Dr. Seymour Diamond, Dr. Mauskop provides this type of computerized relaxation training. He recommends six to eight sessions, usually 30 minutes each once a week, which allows you to learn how to control your body better by teaching you how to relax and not tightening your neck and scalp muscles, and how to breathe regularly. This has been beneficial for both migraine and tension headaches.
- *Supplements.* Research at the New York Headache Center has shown that an intravenous injection of magnesium can result in a dramatic improvement in up to 50 percent of migraine sufferers. The center has a commercial relationship with the manufacturer Natural Science Corporation of America, based in Encino, California, which makes Migra-Lieve. It is a product that combines magnesium, riboflavin, and feverfew, three natural ingredients that have been shown in scientific trials to prevent migraine headaches.

THE DOC'S SUPPLEMENT LIST

According to Dr. Mauskop, research shows that these certain vitamins and minerals may bring headache relief.

Supplement	What It Does
B vitamins	Vitamin B_6 may raise serotonin levels (brain chemicals), which lower headache pain; the brain may need B_{12} to function normally and not be vulnerable to headaches caused by food additives
Feverfew	This herb reduces heat and inflammation in the head area; it contains anti-inflammatory compounds, which reduce enlarged and congested blood vessels in the head
Magnesium	An anti-stress mineral that helps relax the smooth muscles of blood vessels, which lowers risk of headaches and may lessen migraines; it works on neurotransmitter receptors to block pain messages; stress causes your headaches possibly by lowering your magnesium level

Safety Smarts: Feverfew: Do not use for kids younger than 2 or if you are pregnant or breast-feeding.

DR. GULEVICH'S MIGRAINE MAGIC

STEVEN GULEVICH, M.D.

52

Did you know that Botox® injections can be used for wrinkles and headaches? "Botox® works by blocking transmission between nerve ending and muscle. The effect is to partially weaken the injected muscle," explains neurologist Dr. Steven Gulevich, who performs approximately two hundred Botox® injections weekly. "Many wrinkles result from activity of the muscle under the skin, and thus respond to Botox®. This also helps relieve migraine and tension headaches, but we're not sure if that's all."

Botox® is the brand name of botulinum toxin Type A, that has been in use since about 1990. In 2001, botulinum toxin Type B was introduced under the name of Myobloc®. Steven Gulevich, M.D., has experience with both. Both forms of this naturally occurring substance, Botox® and Myobloc®, are injected into muscle that is contracting abnormally. The medications partially weaken the nerve to the muscle for about four to six months. Botox® has proven useful in people who suffer from abnormal contraction of muscle.

Adds Dr. Gulevich, "Some headache medications can constrict some of the blood vessels to the heart and can't be given to people with heart conditions." Botox®, however, is very safe, according to him, and he personally would take a Botox® injection if it were needed.

Doc's Rx to Heal Yourself

- If you have chronic headaches, consult with your doctor to find out whether beta blockers and antidepressants may work for you.
- Consider cognitive therapy and biofeedback to control your headaches.
- B vitamins can help bring headache relief.
- Magnesium can lower your risk of headaches and may lower your risk of migraines.
- Feverfew can help prevent migraines.
- Botox® can help both migraines and tension headaches.

Bios

Seymour Diamond, M.D., a neurologist, is the director of Diamond Headache Clinic in Chicago, established in 1972. He is the coauthor of *Conquering Your Migraine* and *Headaches and Your Child* (both by Simon & Schuster). He received his M.D. degree from the Chicago Medical School in Chicago, Illinois. Dr. Diamond has received the American Headache Society Lifetime Achievement award. At 76, he lives in Chicago, Illinois. He has three daughters and six grandchildren. Web site: www.diamond headache.com.

Steven Gulevich, M.D., is board certified in neurology and electro-diagnostic medicine. He received the doctor of medicine degree from Duke University. At 42, he is a full-time neurologist at the Swedish Hospital at Englewood, Colorado. He is married, has two children, and lives in Englewood.

Alexander Mauskop, M.D., is a board-certified neurologist who went to medical school in the former Soviet Union, is the director of the New York Headache Center, and is an associate professor of clinical neurology at the State University of New York. He is the coauthor of *The Headache Alternative* (Bantam Doubleday Dell Publishing Group) and *What Your Doctor May Not Tell You About Migraines* (Warner Books). He has a practice in New York City, resides in Larchmont, New York, is married, and has two children. Web site: www.nyheadache.com.

22

Insomnia

GETTING *Z*'S WITH DR. BROCH'S TIPS

LAUREN BROCH, PH.D.

American adults sleep, on average, seven hours a night, about an hour less than the eight recommended by sleep experts. While we know that sleep restores and replenishes body and mind, lack of sleep depletes energy, frazzles nerves, and breaks down the immune system. That's where Dr. Lauren Broch, Ph.D., comes in. She helps sleep-deprived people get back to basic bed behavior.

Following is Dr. Broch's five-step plan to get some shut-eye:

1. Keep a sleep log. An important step is to find out what is causing your sleepless nights, says Dr. Broch. So she has people keep a log and write down what time they went to bed, the number of times they awakened during the night, and the number of times they got up.

2. Adjust your bed behavior. "Among the main treatments that have been found to be effective for insomnia are behavioral treatments. I will ask people what they're eating or whether they're eating late at night—that's not going to

help them sleep well," says Dr. Broch, who points out the main culprits, which include caffeine, cola, chocolates, and alcohol.

3. Use bedtime basics. To get adequate *z*'s, Dr. Broch recommends that her patients listen to relaxing music, drink warm cups of herbal tea, experience a soothing massage just before bedtime, and don't use the bedroom for work or worry.

4. Problem-solve during the day. Failure to deal with stress in your day-to-day life can cause sleeplessness. "At night the awake brain will think about the things that are not resolved. So I encourage people to make worry lists so they deal with some of the stresses in their life during the day and attempt to make resolutions," says Dr. Broch.

5. Work out. Exercise in the latter part of the afternoon (but not the evening) seems to be more advantageous because it helps the brain get into a deeper sleep, says Dr. Broch.

Unfortunately, sleeplessness affects all of us at one time or another. Dr. Broch, for instance, told me that when her mother had a stroke it caused the doctor high anxiety. Her temporary sleeping difficulty was compounded by her menstrual cycle, so that about a week before her period, she was having much more insomnia. To cope, she turned to her own natural strategies to help get better sleep. She also included deep breathing exercises and yoga.

DOC'S RX TO HEAL YOURSELF

- Keep a sleep log to determine what is causing your sleepless nights.
- Avoid sleep thieves such as cola, chocolate, caffeine, and alcohol.
- Try soothing herbal teas and massage before bedtime.
- Problem-solve during the day, and be happy and don't worry at night.

Bio

Lauren Broch, PH.D., received her degree in psychology at the City College of the City University of New York in New York City. She is a 42-year-old director of education and training at the New York–Presbyterian Hospital Sleep-Wake Disorders Center in White Plains, New York. She lives in Rybrook, New York, is married, and has two children.

23

Stress

DR. FRY'S LAUGH-MORE METHOD

WILLIAM F. FRY, M.D.

Dr. William Fry claims that universal humor, such as laughing during the best and worst of times (which can and does hit everyone), is the kind that connects us and helps to relax us.

"Humor and laughter are infectious," says laughter expert Dr. Fry. And if you learn what tickles your funny bone, whether it be reading the funny pages or watching *I Love Lucy* reruns, you can join Dr. Fry. He is a jovial man with an upbeat attitude, and gets his daily dose of good and destressing belly laughs. Here's how to laugh yourself mellow.

- Humor beats anxiety. Ever notice how sharing jokes in TV sitcoms like *Mad About You* helps the couple to lighten up during life's ups and downs? You can bet Dr. Fry, an even-tempered senior, reaps the health benefits of this same type of good humor in his own family matters, which consist of a spouse, grown kids and grandchildren.
- Humor lessens stressors. Let's face it. People who have a good sense of humor, like Dr. Fry does, can cope better with

stressful situations. In fact, laughter is a super way to release pent-up anger, which has been linked to heart disease. Indeed, the good doctor knows that looking for the silliness in life can help you to deal with problems.

Dr. Fry reminded me (I have interviewed him before) of a touching letter from a veteran who survived the D-Day invasion. And because just one trooper made a joke, it helped to release tension and provided a temporary and destressing escape for everyone.

- Humor accepts aging woes. Ever notice how some folks don't take life's aging process too seriously (despite enduring an awkward senior moment)? Dr. Fry (almost 80) believes we all should laugh more—like he does—for better health. And it's free.

DR. BORYSENKO'S TIME-OUT

JOAN BORYSENKO, PH.D.

Dr. Joan Borysenko, former director of the Mind/Body Clinic at two different Harvard teaching hospitals and author of *Inner Peace for Busy People* (Hay House), says: "Somewhere between 70 and 90 percent of visits to family practice physicians are due to stress. And stress can make almost any illness worse."

So what does the busy anti-stress doctor do today to head off stress and find inner peace? "For me it's a continuing journey. Because it's so easy for all the good things you know to get swept aside when life is so busy. Particularly in my case because I travel 150 days a year. What I'm trying to do in my own life is to find ways that will help keep my body, mind, and spirit in the best condition that don't take hours every day," she says. Here are some of her latest findings:

- *Finding balance is a myth.* "Sometimes you have an enormous project and everything else is going to have to be on hold while you work on that for a month. Other times the children are sick. Everything else has to go on hold for that priority," explains Dr. Borysenko. So in an imperfect world, forget trying to achieve perfect balance, because it's not going to happen.

- *Listen to your body.* "If you give up those things like working out when your body is asking for it, you're going to find that all the tasks you have to do will not get done as well as they would if you take that time first for yourself," she says. "If you don't listen to your body, you're going to end up stressed at the end of the day."
- *Avoid burnout.* "In our society, because we are so busy and pay so little attention to ourselves, most people are working in the slightly overwhelmed mode. So they're still getting a lot done, but they're burning their body out. They're stressed, they're starting to get anxious. Once you're in the overwhelmed mode, that's when people tend to ignore themselves entirely and say, 'Oh, I don't have time to work out,' and, 'I don't have time to eat right.'
- *Take care of yourself first.* "What I'm trying to teach people is, if you take the time to treat yourself better, you'll actually shift to the left on that stress productivity curve. You'll be less stressed and you'll get more done. So taking care of yourself actually helps you to be more productive and creative."

HOW DR. BORYSENKO CHILLS OUT

Check out how the lucky doc takes time to smell the flowers of life:

- "I live in the mountains. I really enjoy getting outside and hiking or gardening."
- "I love to watch the wildlife. I watch the birds and deer. I find just sitting on the deck and watching nature to be a very important thing."

- "I meditate five or ten minutes a day and I often do it out in the hot tub."
- "I have a very nice cuddly husband."
- "And I'm always cuddling my dogs—that's why we have four of them (a collie, miniature schnauzer, Maltese, and shih tzu)—which provides soothing touch therapy, a wonderful destressor."

GRR-EAT STRESS REDUCERS FOR DR. COREN

STANLEY COREN, PH.D.

One thing that bonded my father and me was dogs. Dr. Coren, a devout dog person, reminds me of my late dad. Both men value dogs. And I discovered that dogs do more for this doctor than just provide canine cuddles.

"Two dogs that I have in my life at the moment are a flat-coated retriever named Odin, 4, and a Nova Scotia duck-tolling retriever, Dancer, 2. They are my excuse to get out of the house twice a day. When I'm writing books I become incredibly focused on what I'm doing. But I've got to do something to clear my mind, because otherwise I'm going to go to bed at night and dream the work. Instead of resting I'll be moving paragraphs in my sleep," he told me, and as an author always on deadline I could totally relate.

To remedy working 24/7, Dr. Coren walks the dogs at night. "It's the very last thing I do to wind down. The thing about it is I get to watch them move. We're just walking along, keeping pace with each other, and the mind sort of just shuts off. By the time I get back, things have cleared," he says.

"A lot of the research has been done by Alan Beck. What he and his associates have been able to show is that if you pet a familiar dog, a whole bunch of physiological changes will occur. For example, your breathing becomes deeper and slower. Your heartbeat slows and your muscles relax. In other words, you show all the signs of reduced tension."

"For me," adds Dr. Coren, "I sometimes very consciously use my dogs to destress. If I'm having a rough time, for example. If they recycle years, this is not a year that I want to recycle. I've lost four family members in the last two months including my mother and an aunt who helped raise me when my father was in the army and overseas. The big problem here, in the family setting, is that I'm supposed to be providing strength for other individuals," he laughs. "I'm the psychologist, and therefore I'm bombproof, right? My father had been married to my mother for 61 years and he really needed a lot of support. That meant that I could not make demands on other family members and I had to be strong," says Dr. Coren.

So the Rock of Gibraltar doctor turned to his dogs for comfort. "And the thing of it is that they empathize. They pick up that something is wrong and they will come and snuggle up to you. So that really works," says Dr. Coren. In fact, he concludes, "What's keeping my dad sane, having lost my mother, is the fact that he's got a 12-year-old Cavalier King Charles spaniel named Amy. He talks to her all the time, takes her with him every place."

Adds Dr. Coren, "Another way of destressing is when you're in a social situation where you just don't like what's going on. I will say, 'Well, I'd really like to stay and finish discussing this, but I have to work with my dogs because we're going into competition in a week or two.' And all of sudden I'm out of the situation," he says and laughs in his easygoing style.

"It's an interesting thing, because the mind of the dog is like the mind of a 2-year-old. But they're so athletic. They're so absolutely beautiful and you watch them. It's an aesthetic experience. For them it's the way they get in tune to the universe and it's the equivalent of dancing," says Dr. Coren. He concludes, "There are times when I feel out of sorts and I take the dogs out and throw something for them to go after and they take off and start to run and I say, "Yes! There is god!"

RESEARCH IN A NUTSHELL

People in the company of a dog, not unlike Dr. Coren, are more apt to be viewed by others as friendlier, happier, and more relaxed than people who are dogless. ("The influence of animals on social perception," in Beck, Alan, and Katcher, Aaron (eds.), *New Perspectives on Our Lives with Companion Animals* (Philadelphia: University of Pennsylvania Press, 1983), pp. 64–71)

FACTS F.Y.I

American Animal Hospital Association 2000 Pet Owner Survey:

- Nearly 29 percent of the 1,189 respondents rely on their pet the most for companionship and affection.
- 48 percent of singles rely on their pets the most for companionship and affection.
- 80 percent of dog owners take their canines along on errands.

DOCS' RX TO HEAL YOURSELF

- Laugh more.
- Go back to nature to destress and reconnect with yourself and the world.
- Take control of your life.
- Savor intimate relationships.
- Go to the dogs for a naturally calming fix.

BIOS

Joan Borysenko, Ph.D., went to the Division of Medical Sciences, where she got her Ph.D. at the Harvard Medical School in

Boston, Massachusetts. At 55, she is the author of ten books including *Meditation as Medicine* (Pocket Books). She is married, has two children and four stepchildren, and lives in Boulder, Colorado. Web site: joanborysenko.com.

Stanley Coren, Ph.D., is a professor in the Department of Psychology at the University of British Columbia. He did his undergraduate work at the University of Pennsylvania and completed his doctorate in psychology at Stanford. He is the author of bestselling books on dogs, such as *How to Speak Dog* and *Why We Love the Dogs We Do* (both by Free Press). He lives in Vancouver, British Columbia, is 59, is married, and has two children. Web site: Stanleycoren.com.

William F. Fry, M.D., is associate professor emeritus of Stanford University in Palo Alto, California. He received his medical degree at the University of Cincinnati, Ohio. At 77, he is retired and has three children and six grandchildren. He resides in Nevada City, California, with his wife.

PART VI

The Female Body

My friend Helen told me one day about her breast cancer night-mare. One fall day 30 years ago, when she was a kindergartner, Helen waved to her pretty, teary-eyed 42-year-old mommy inside a hospital room. Her mother had just undergone a radical mastectomy.

Two months later, her only aunt, at 39, was diagnosed with breast cancer, too. Years later, her kindhearted grandmother developed the same disease at 82.

Today, even though her relatives survived breast cancer, the 36-year-old native northern Californian, a busy mom and part-time state park ranger, fears getting the malady that can kill. Although Helen is at higher risk, no woman is immune.

But she knows—like the woman doctors in Part VI, "The Female Body,"—how by changing your diet and certain risk factors, not only can help you save your breasts and your life, but you can lessen other female woes, from premenstrual syndrome (PMS) to the hormonal changes (from perimenopause to menopause).

Women's health specialist Dr. Heather Pena, M.D., shares her personal immunity-boosting nutrition plan to lower your risk of breast cancer.

Susan Lark, M.D., another doctor who is well known for her

books on preventive care and women's health, discusses how she fought the battle against PMS and found the cure, naturally.

And Drs. Joyce Kaakis and Carolyn DeMarco discuss their woman-to-woman strategies in dealing with perimenopause and menopause.

24

Breast Cancer

Dr. Pena's Health Protection Plan

HEATHER PENA, M.D.

Breast cancer: the statistics are sobering. One in eight women will contract this disease. But as frightening as this may seem, we're not powerless. We don't have to wait for fate to randomly deal us a bad hand. There *are* steps we can take to lower our risk. And one of the most important is to adopt a cancer-fighting diet.

To help you determine the best anti–breast cancer diet strategy, I consulted with Heather Pena, M.D., formerly of the Pritikin Longevity Center in Santa Monica, California. She understands the threat of this deadly dilemma. Here, she shares the basis for her disease-fighting diet.

FACTS F.Y.I.

According to the American Cancer Society:

- Breast cancer is second only to lung cancer in cancer deaths in women.

- An estimated 205,000 men and women are expected to have breast cancer in the year 2002 in the United States.
- About 40,000 breast cancer victims will die in 2002.
- The epidemic strikes in urban areas hardest, although the reason is still unknown.

CUT FAT TO 20 PERCENT

Research has pointed to a cancer-fat connection. Says Dr. Pena, "There is some evidence in populations in the world whose diets are 20 percent or less from fat that they have a lower incidence of breast cancer. For example, the Japanese have among the lowest rates of breast cancer in the world."

One reason dietary fat may contribute to cancer is its link to the production of estrogen, a female hormone. Women whose diets are high in fat tend to have more estrogen circulating in their bloodstream that may cause a mutation in the cells in the breasts, which may encourage the growth of tumors, she explains.

"When you're eating a high-fat diet or you're overweight, you have too much estrogen. But with a diet like Dr. Pena's (at 5'5" she maintains a healthy weight at 125 pounds), estrogen levels normalize and go down to a more ideal range.

EAT MORE VEGETABLES

Follow the National Cancer Institute's (NCI) guidelines to eat five or more servings of fruits and vegetables a day—especially vegetables from the cabbage family, such as broccoli, cauliflower, and brussels sprouts.

"There is some evidence that a chemical called indole carbinol found in these cruciferous vegetables helps to decrease levels of the bad estrogen," says Dr. Pena, who makes it a point to get crucifers such as cauliflower and cabbage daily. The bad estrogen may cause a mutation in the cells of the breasts that triggers the production of tumors. The good estrogen helps keep our bones strong and our skin supple.

And, she adds, anything that balances the ratio of the "bad" estrogen and the "good" estrogen in the body seems to decrease the risk of developing breast cancer. Indoles, which you get from the cruciferous vegetables and soy, have been shown to do that. Dr. Pena eats 20 to 40 grams of soy per day from tofu, soybeans, and soy milk (½ cup is about 20 grams of soy protein) and flaxseed (a health food that is a good source of omega-3 oils, which contain isoflavones and lignans, which may guard against hormone-related cancers).

In addition, for an alternative cancer-fighting breakfast, Dr. Pena whips up a healthful shake: nonfat milk or soy milk fortified with calcium, frozen blueberries and strawberries, 1 tablespoon of flaxseed, and a handful of raw oatmeal.

Sample One-Day Cancer-Fighting Diet Plan

Breakfast: Oatmeal topped with skim milk and berries.

Snack: Fruit or low-sodium vegetable soup.

Lunch: Vegetable salad. Low-fat vegetarian burrito.

Snack: Corn or artichoke or lentil salad.

Dinner: Chicken, fish, or pasta. Vegetables (two or three). Skim milk or green tea.

Snack: Fresh fruit or nonfat yogurt. Skim milk or green tea.

Boost Your Fiber Intake

For added breast cancer protection, Dr. Pena combines a low-fat diet with high-fiber foods. "The best sources are fruits, vegetables, and whole grains. That's also been shown to be protective. What's interesting, the flaxseed fiber (called the lignan) has also shown

protective effects against breast cancer," says Dr. Pena, who con-
sumes 40 to 50 grams of fiber each day.

To lower your risk of cancer, the National Cancer Institute
recommends you increase your fiber intake to between 20 and 30
grams a day by eating a variety of fiber-rich foods. Just ½ cup of
canned chickpeas has 7 grams of fiber; 1 ounce of bran cereal (⅓
cup) has 10.

WATCH YOUR ALCOHOL INTAKE

Alcohol may increase the production of estrogen in the body,
says Dr. Pena, thereby increasing your risk of cancer. While the
jury is still out on exactly how much alcohol increases breast cancer risk, follow Dr. Pena's recommendation (she drinks only a
glass of wine a couple of times a month) and drinks alcohol in
moderation if at all.

KEEP YOUR LIFESTYLE HEALTHY

Exercise has been shown to be protective against breast cancer, says Dr. Pena. While the reason is unknown, Dr. Pena specu-
lates that exercise may affect the ratio of "good" to "bad"
estrogen. Meanwhile, Dr. Pena walks at least three days a week—
thirty to forty-five minutes each time—on the treadmill.

While a healthy diet and staying physically active are important, so is early breast cancer detection. And Dr. Pena is well
aware of the self-help strategies.

Warning signs can vary from an abnormality on a mammogram to breast changes such as a lump, thickening, swelling, dim-
pling, skin irritation, distortion, scaliness, and pain or tenderness.

Mammograms will detect about 90 percent of the breast cancers of women without symptoms. They are somewhat more ac-
curate in postmenopausal women than premenopausal women.
The American Cancer Society recommends mammograms every
year for women age 40 and older. Consult with your doctor be-

cause frequency may depend on your family history of cancer and other risk factors.

And note, a breast self-exam is recommended once a month. It's best to do it about one week after your period, when your breasts are not tender to the touch.

Doc's Rx to Heal Yourself

- Eat a low-fat diet to keep your estrogen levels normal.
- Consume vegetables, especially crucifers, to balance the good and bad estrogen in your body.
- Opt for more fiber in your daily diet to protect against cancer.
- Limit your intake of alcohol, because it may increase estrogen and raise your odds of developing breast cancer.
- Exercise regularly because, it may help provide extra protection to balance the estrogen ratio in your body.
- Get a physical checkup, and do monthly self breast exams. Discuss with your health practitioner when and how often you should get a mammogram.

Bio

Heather Pena, M.D., is an internist specializing in preventive medicine and women's health. She is a graduate of Tufts University, where she received her bachelor of science in Biology. Dr. Pena graduated from Harvard Medical School. She is on the staff at Santa Monica–UCLA Hospital and St. John's Hospital. At 45, she is married and has a son.

25

Menstrual Problems

Dr. Lark's PMS Diet

SUSAN LARK, M.D.

Dr. Susan Lark remembers the scourge of premenstrual syndrome (PMS), a disorder of the female hormone system. "As a teenager I had a lot of unpleasant symptoms, bloating, food cravings, and acne and oily skin—and I became aware of mood swings as I got a little older," she told me.

"During medical school I had both PMS and cramps. The last couple of years I was sometimes on call all night taking care of patients. And the days were incredibly long and difficult. I often compare it to going to Marine boot camp. I remember having incredibly severe cramps so that I'd have to leave work and go to the on-call room and just sit there in misery."

Dr. Lark adds, "My PMS went on forever, up to ten days to two weeks at a time. I really had bad PMS. I tried everything during medical school. I had good teachers and doctors that I worked with who put me on pain pills, birth control pills, and all kinds of anti-inflammatories. But nothing really helped."

It wasn't until her first year of postgraduate training that Dr.

Lark read an article on nutrition and female-related issues. She became interested in complementary therapies such as stress reduction that were linked to improving health. She started to practice biofeedback and yoga and modified her diet, stopped eating a lot of junk food, and found that her PMS became increasingly better.

To fight the monthly malaise, women, first and foremost, need to take a diet approach, says Dr. Lark, who wrote the *PMS Self Help Book* (Celestial Arts).

All the ingredients that can help reduce or prevent premenstrual syndrome (PMS) can be found in the kitchen. Sound absurd? Well, it's not. Certain foods can affect cramps, irritability, and food cravings for better or for worse.

At least 150 symptoms (which occur before menstruation) have been linked to PMS, including bloating, weight gain, nervous tension, mood swings, breast tenderness, irritability, depression, headaches, and increased appetite.

While one-third to one-half of all women may experience PMS during their reproductive years (even up to 90 percent may have very mild symptoms), the exact cause of PMS is still unknown. It is known that women who eat an unhealthy diet can exacerbate symptoms. But there is an antidote to break the cycle of PMS, says Dr. Lark: eating right.

THE DOC'S PMS FOOD LIST

A diet rich in vitamins and minerals found in foods can provide PMS relief. Here are Dr. Lark's suggested PMS food cures:

PMS Symptoms	Food Cures	What They Do
Cramps and pain	Collard leaves, salmon, shrimp, sesame seeds, and broccoli	Provide calcium, which may prevent cramps and pain

Premenstrual acne and oily skin	Carrots, butternut squash, salmon, dandelion greens, and sweet potatoes	Provide vitamin A, which can stave off acne and oily skin
Irritability, mood swings, fluid retention, breast tenderness, bloating, sugar craving, and fatigue	Salmon, chicken, tuna, and soybeans	Provide vitamin B, which can help ward off irritability, mood swings, fluid retention, breast tenderness, bloating, sugar cravings, and fatigue
Stress	Sweet red peppers, collard greens, kale, strawberries, oranges, and grapefruit	Provide vitamin C, which fights stress
Anxiety, irritability, depression, food cravings	Wheat germ, apples, turnip greens, brussels sprouts, and sweet potatoes	Provide vitamin E, which can reduce anxiety, irritability, despression, and food cravings
Moodiness, acne	Chicken, rice bran, black-eyed peas, and garbanzos	Provide zinc, which can help control acne and counterbalance copper, which can regulate moodiness and estrogen levels
Menstrual cramps	Soybeans, beet greens, shrimp, salmon, and tofu	Provide magnesium, which aids in calcium absorption and soothes menstrual cramps
Fluid retention and bloating	Fruit, vegetables, seeds, and nuts	Provide potassium, which may help reduce fluid retention and bloating

WHICH FOODS SHOULD BE SKIPPED?

Many of the foods women crave when feeling the menstrual blues are a woman's worst enemy. Dr. Lark knows PMS patients often binge on chocolate and sweets, which can result not only in sugar "lows," but also in weight gain.

To counteract sweet cravings, women should eat unsweetened carob instead of chocolate, suggests Dr. Lark. It's nutritious and high in calcium. They can also try honey instead of sugar. It's two and a half times as sweet and won't intensify sugar blues or sugar cravings.

"All caffeine beverages and foods, fruit juice, alcohol, and refined sugar aggravate PMS symptoms terribly," says Dr. Lark.

Other foods to add to the PMS hit list? Salt, dairy products, and red meat. These foods can contribute to a variety of PMS symptoms, from bloating to breast tenderness.

PMS sufferers will discover that, if handled with a positive attitude, a healthy balanced diet—along with exercise, relaxation, and the use of vitamin and mineral supplements—can help win the battle against PMS naturally.

THE DOC'S SUPPLEMENT LIST

Some of the supplements Dr. Lark used to prevent PMS symptoms and then found that they helped some of her patients included these three vitamins.

Supplement	What It Does
Vitamin E	Vitamin E can help reduce anxiety, irritability, depression, and food cravings. It can also lessen PMS-related breast tenderness.
Vitamin B complex	The vitamin B complex can help remedy the irritability that result when emotional stress causes loss of water-soluble B vitamins from the body.

| Vitamin C | "Vitamin C is an important antioxidant and anti-stress vitamin. It is necessary for immune function. It also has an antihistamine effect, which can help women whose allergies worsen before their periods," says Dr. Lark. |

Safety Smarts: Vitamin C: If you take too much, it can cause gastrointestinal problems.

DOC'S RX TO HEAL YOURSELF

- Eat a low-fat diet rich in vitamins and minerals.
- Stay clear of culprits such as chocolate, caffeine, fruit juice, and refined sugar that worsen PMS symptoms.
- Avoid salt, dairy products, and red meat, which can make bloating worse.
- Take vitamin B complex and antioxidant vitamins C and E to help reduce PMS symptoms.
- Opt for destressing techniques to cope with anxiety and depression.

BIO

Susan Lark, M.D., a 55-year-old physician-educator who is a well-known authority in the fields of clinical nutrition and preventive medicine, has written nine books on women's health issues. A graduate of Northwestern University Medical School, she has served on the clinical faculty at Stanford University Medical School in Palo Alto, California, where she continues to teach in the division of Family and Community Medicine. She is married and lives in Los Altos, California. To subscribe to *The Lark Letter/Daily Balance,* go to www.phillips.com/health/catalog.htm or www.drlark.com.

26

Perimenopause

Dr. DeMarco's Perimenopause Pointers

CAROLYN DEMARCO, M.D.

59

Surprise! Women not only have menopause to deal with, they also can get a wake-up call with perimenopause—the period before your period stops. Dr. Carolyn DeMarco, author of *Take Charge of Your Body: Women's Health Advisor* (Well Women Press), told me that she is perimenopausal.

Symptoms can vary from woman to woman. However, they can include anxiety, skipped periods, mood swings, weight gain, and insomnia. Not only does Dr. DeMarco treat patients and friends in this stage of life, but she also treats herself.

SHUT-EYE, HORMONAL BALANCE, AND PEACE

The fact is, sleep problems may be a problem for many perimenopausal women. This can be due to hot flashes, anxiety, and depression. "Women function during the day better, with more clarity and calmness, when they have had seven to eight hours of sleep," explains Dr. DeMarco. And she sees to it that she gets adequate shut-eye.

"Especially in the perimenopause," she told me, "getting a good night's sleep is one of my top health priorities. I sleep in a room with many windows, with only natural light, including moonlight. I sleep on a good mattress, with a special magnetic mattress underneath. The magnetic mattress simulates the earth's magnetic field, which has been steadily declining. So the effect of the mattress is to help me sleep more deeply and recover more quickly from the wear and tear of the day."

In addition to getting adequate sleep, Dr. DeMarco uses a natural progesterone cream to balance her hormones and to prevent bone loss. She applies the cream on rotating sites on the skin from day 12 to 26 as she is still menstruating; after menopause she will use it 21 to 25 days of every month.

Dr. DeMarco also frequently applies to her skin high-quality therapeutic-grade essential oils like lavender, sandalwood, frankincense, geranium, and rosewood and special blends like Joy, Peace, and Calming.

REVVING UP THE IMMUNE SYSTEM

During the perimenopause years, Dr. DeMarco believes the most important preventive measure is to power up the immune system so it will be ready for action to attack both infectious invaders and cancer cells. Other culprits include stressors such as radiation, noise, chlorinated water, smog, and depleted and chemical-laden food.

The best approach, says Dr. DeMarco, is "a new blend of plant sterols and sterolins known as Moducare. Excellent-quality research on human subjects shows Moducare enhances the natural killer cells that fight viruses, fungi, bacteria, and cancer cells. At the same time, Moducare decreases the type of T-cells that cause inflammation and orchestrate the autoimmune attack."

A perimenopause bonus: Moducare helps to balance the adrenal gland by decreasing the stress hormone cortisol and increasing the master adrenal hormone DHEA.

THE DOC'S SUPPLEMENT LIST

Here are some of the supplements Dr. DeMarco takes to make the transitional years easier.

Supplement	What It Does	Dose
Vitamin C	An antioxidant that prevents cancer and heart disease	500 mg
Tryptophan	An essential amino acid that helps promote better sleep and prevent insomnia	200 mg
Magnesium citrate	Promotes bone health, calms nerves, lessens stress on the heart, and enhances sleep	300 mg
Herbal bowel cleanser	Cleanses the colon and gets rid of toxins that accumulate daily	

Safety Smarts: If you take too much vitamin C, it can cause gastrointestinal problems.

BEATING THE PESKY PAUSE WITH DR. GITTLEMAN

ANN LOUISE GITTLEMAN, N.D.

For countless women, perimenopausal symptoms can be more annoying and frightening than both PMS and menopause combined. Dr. Ann Louise Gittleman told me in her own words how she solved the problem naturally:

Many years ago, after several sleepless nights, I was once again wide awake at 3:00 A.M. with heart palpitations. I began to seriously wonder if this was the beginning of a heart condition or some kind of a nervous breakdown. Something was definitely changing in my 40-something body, and I began to imagine the possibility of never sleeping through the night again, causing me to become even more anxious and depressed.

It wasn't until I took a FSH [follicle-stimulating hormone] test that it dawned on me what was really happening. I wasn't going crazy. I had entered the perimenopause zone—a life cycle change of about ten years during which the body shifts its output and handling of the hormones needed for reproduction. Interestingly, over the past ten years, I had definitely become more irritable and less patient, with a shorter fuse and a shortened attention span. I simply attributed these personality changes to my increased focus on work. It never once occurred to me that something biochemical, like hormones, was changing in my body and affecting my brain and nervous system. Besides, I didn't have any of the other telltale symptoms like hot flashes or night sweats that were common signals of mid-life fluctuations.

Perimenopause is no longer "the PMS from hell." Based upon my experience and supported by current research studies, I set out to find a natural remedy that would set me straight. I kept reading about the benefits of high-lignan flaxseed oil for perimenopausal women like me. And then I reviewed my files again and learned that many of my own clients use evening primrose oil (a woman's botanical oil) to overcome their symptoms. So I started combining a couple of tablespoons of the flaxseed oil with evening primrose oil supplements on a daily basis and found that in less than a week I was calmer, more focused, and even sleeping through the night.

THE DOC'S SUPPLEMENT LIST

Dr. Gittleman gets these two supplements in a combination product; however, some women can and do take them separately.

Supplement	What It Does
Flaxseed oil	This high-lignan oil component relieves depression, fatigue, and allergies, but the lignans themselves are estrogenlike substances that have balancing effects on serotonin and other mood regulators
Evening primrose oil	This oil is beneficial for fighting irritability, mood changes, anxiety, fluid retention, and even sleep disorders

DOC'S RX TO HEAL YOURSELF

- Get adequate shut-eye, which can help lessen perimenopausal problems.
- Boost your immune system with the plant sterols found in Moducare, which help during perimenopausal years to stay healthy and prevent age-related diseases.
- Take your supplements—vitamin C, tryptophan, and magnesium citrate, which can help enhance your body during the perimenopausal years.
- Consider taking flaxseed oil, evening primrose oil, and soy isoflavones to prevent a variety of perimenopausal symptoms.

BIOS

Carolyn DeMarco, M.D., graduated from the University of Toronto. She is a general practitioner with a special interest in women's health and alternative medicine. Dr. DeMarco has a CD-ROM entitled *Everything You Wanted to Know About Women*. She is the author of *Take Charge of Your Body* (Well Women Press). At 53, she resides in British Columbia.

Ann Louise Gittleman, N.D., received her N.D. degree at Bernadean University, Van Nuys, California. She writes, teaches, and lectures both nationally and internationally. She consults with patients on a limited basis. She is the author of *Before the Change: Taking Charge of Your Perimenopause* (Harper-SanFrancisco) and *The Fat Flush Plan* (McGraw-Hill). She lives in Bozeman, Montana, has a "significant other," and has two nephews, one niece, and a surrogate daughter. Web site: www.annlouise.com.

27

Menopause

MAKING SUBTLE CHANGES WITH DR. KAAKIS

JOYCE KAAKIS, M.D.

Dr. Joyce Kaakis is a gynecologist whom plenty of women would love to have as their own doctor for female-related problems. Interestingly, she says that 80 percent of her patients are either perimenopausal or menopausal.

By seeing women, day after day, who have the common complaints (hot flashes or "temperature disturbances," depression, irritability, and mood swings), is it frightening for the doctor when The Change is right around the corner for herself?

Not really. She's got a handle on both natural and traditional hormone therapy—creams, gels, pills, and patches to suit each individual woman's needs—including her own when The Change arrives.

THE CHANGES

"My definition of menopause is when you have PMS [premenstrual syndrome] all month long. PMS is very much like menopause except that it tends to be only ten days before your period. As you get closer to menopause, it gets more severe," explains Dr. Kaakis.

At 44, Dr. Kaakis is starting to see a change in her own menstrual cycle. "Most women who say they haven't experienced any change are often too busy to notice. But I think the average person sees a change somewhere between 42 and 45," she says.

When I told the doctor that at 48, I still have regular periods but my PMS symptoms seem to be worse she shot back, "Have you had your hormone levels assessed?" "No," I answered. So I asked her, "What hormone tests?" "The FSH [follicle-stimulating hormone] and estradiol [a hormone] together as a pair." "Why would I want to do that?" I retorted.

"Because those are the two markers of your pituitary gland and your ovaries and predict if failure is starting," Dr. Kaakis explains. And the reason that you want to know sooner than later is that if you are prone to osteoporosis and heart disease, you don't want to go several years without protection. "And for those people who are not very symptomatic and don't have any risk factors, it's a point of information—a baseline. So then later when you have to make decisions you can repeat them," she adds.

Has Dr. Kaakis had her hormone levels checked? Yes indeed, she says. "So what I know for a fact is that my levels are still normal, but I'm starting to have some of the cyclic changes. Not everybody goes through the same order. In some people the period is the last thing to go. Everything else starts happening first. In some people it's the first thing to get screwed up: in terms of bleeding, irregularity, more frequent or less frequent. In some people the mood is the first thing to go: You'll start having more depression and irritability. And the labs do not always change as soon as the trouble starts. So they're just one factor. But they need to be checked because if it's unclear, sometimes they help clarify what the situation is."

Keep in mind, adds Dr. Kaakis, it's important to find the right doctor for you. "Of course, the bottom line is competence. However, you want someone you get along with. Because if you don't, you're not going to share your personal feelings and things that are bothering you in the way you need to."

FACTS F.Y.I.

- According to the North American Menopause Society (NAMS), the average age of spontaneous menopause is 51, but it can take place in your thirties or sixties.
- The time leading up to menopause, perimenopause, starts about age 47.
- "It has been estimated that 75 to 80 percent of women passing through menopause experience one or more symptoms, but only 10 to 35 percent are affected strongly enough to see professional help," says Linda Ojeda, Ph.D., in her book *Menopause Without Medicine* (Hunter House).
- FSH levels greater than 30 are common for postmenopausal women, according to *Could It Be . . . Perimenopause?* by Steven R. Goldstein, M.D., and Laurie Ashner (Little, Brown and Company).

ESTROGEN THERAPY

What does Dr. Kaakis recommend? "Both personally and when I'm treating patients and family, I start with natural products. And I don't mean natural over-the-counter. I mean either animal- or plant-based estrogens as opposed to manufactured. Now that doesn't mean I never use those—that's just where I start. Some people do well with Premarin, for example," she says.

"All estrogens have the theoretical potential of increasing breast cancer slightly. It's only slight," she says. "It's a risk-benefit thing. It's not so much Premarin versus any other estrogen. It's estrogen versus no estrogen." She adds, "There are a lot of women who are afraid of taking estrogen because of personal experience with The Pill and some bad press."

THERAPY FOR HOT FLASHES

Dr. Kaakis told me that she will take estrogen therapy when she needs it. How will she know when the time is right? "If I start having symptoms (hot flashes, night sweats) that are interfering with the quality of my life."

Nobody has satisfactorily explained the cause of hot flashes. Diminished levels of estrogen and extra supplies of the hormones FSH (follicle-stimulating hormone) and LH (luteinizing hormone) may play a role.

Personally, Dr. Kaakis is starting to include soybeans in her diet. Some medical experts believe soy may ease menopausal discomfort. This plant contains phytoestrogens, called isoflavones. In some Asian countries, where women consume plenty of soy, hot flashes are all but unknown.

Also, eating a fiber-rich diet can help promote the excretion of estrogen, too. It can lower your risk of breast cancer, heart disease, and weight gain—potential problems during menopause. And that's why Dr. Kaakis eats fruits, vegetables, grains, and soy to ensure fiber protection.

If you want to eat more than phytoestrogen-rich soy, here are some other foods that contain phytoestrogens to add to your daily diet: apples, asparagus, beans, blackberries, carrots, cherries, corn, dried seaweed, flaxseed, garlic, green pepper, oat bran, olive oil, onions, pears, squash, sunflower seeds, wheat germ, and yams.

STAYING ACTIVE

While plant-based estrogen foods can help control menopausal symptoms, you can also exercise, as Dr. Kaakis does. Aerobic activity such as walking, which Dr. Kaakis does twice daily, help lower FSH and LH levels. It helps aid the estrogens you are making to work better, she adds. And it reduces stress on your body that gobbles up your hormones. So when you're in the transition, it'll help.

So what are the chances that Dr. Kaakis and plenty of other women, like you and me, will sail through The Change and have no noticeable changes? "Five percent," she answers. "You'll still get bone loss."

Doc's Rx to Heal Yourself

- Get your hormonal levels checked so you can make diet and lifestyle changes to ease the transition.
- Consider taking natural plant-based estrogens for menopausal changes.
- A soy- and fiber-enriched diet can help with estrogen loss during the menopausal years.
- Exercise may help the estrogen you're still making work more efficiently.

Bio

Joyce Kaakis, M.D., is a Fellow of the American College of Obstetricians and Gynecologists, assistant professor of Obstetrics and Gynecology at the University of California at Irvine College of Medicine, and a nationally acclaimed educator, author, and expert on women's health. She is 44, is married, and lives in Long Beach, California. For more information call 562-799-7975 Web site: Estrogenevangelist.com.

PART VII

The Male Body

At 70, my father worked part-time and played golf regularly; at 74, a friend of mine enjoyed his family ties; and at 80, my next-door neighbor spent time helping others. These men all lived long and fruitful lives.

Most of us know that women, on average, live longer and healthier lives than men. But according to new research, men are starting to catch up to women in their life expectancy.

More men are aging gracefully. They are living longer and healthier lives by avoiding alcohol, tobacco, and drugs. In addition, having a loving spouse and healthy eating habits may also contribute to a healthier male body.

But how can you get on the right track? Here are two male doctors in Part VII, "The Male Body," who candidly discuss ways men can beat the longevity odds through positive living.

Dr. Stephen Strum, M.D., a medical oncologist and director of the Prostate Medical Research Center in Los Angeles, California, states: "I believe that we can learn much about prostate cancer through our understanding of the hormonal pathways in man." He reports the problems and solutions of male menopause, which is intriguing to both men and women. And Allan Magaziner, D.O., one of the nation's leading authorities in nutritional, preventive, and environmental medicine, tells an inspirational story about his father, whom he helped fight the battle against "big P"—prostate cancer.

Included in this section are tips on diet, supplements, and lifestyle changes for men's health. The key to a healthy male body, according to these doctors, is to find the method that works best for you.

28

Prostate Problems

DR. STRUM SPEAKS OUT FOR MEN

STEPHEN STRUM, M.D.

These days it's not uncommon for women to chat frankly about PMS and menopause. But you hardly ever hear a man discussing problems with their body's changes and hormonal stuff.

Dr. Stephen Strum, an oncologist, understands that the male reproductive system is a big deal to the quality of life of men in many ways. First, in the anatomy of the genitourinary (GU) system, we see the very real issues of problems with urine flow occurring as men age. Second, all body systems are affected by declining levels of male hormones or by imbalances of male and female hormones. Third, sexual drive and function are major issues for most men and can affect their quality of life. And finally, male fertility is associated with a healthy GU system.

So why are prostate problems haunting men more than ever in the twenty-first century? "Men are living longer today than in past decades. Imbalance in testosterone and estrogen may well be a significant factor in benign prostatic hyperplasia (BPH)," explains Dr. Strum. (At around age 45, the number of cells in the prostate gland starts to increase, which causes a noncancerous process known as BPH.)

"In addition," he adds, "our lives are more sedentary. This compounds dietary changes leading to increased obesity. Our life is also more stressful, and increased stress and age are associated with declining amounts of male hormones such as DHEA" (dehydroepiandrosterone, which revs up sex drive and can stall the aging process).

MAINTAINING A HEALTHY PROSTATE

If symptoms of BPH are mild or nonexistent, the prevention path is a good one to take. By following Dr. Strum's personal dietary strategies you can help balance your hormones, stave off prostate problems, and improve your well-being.

- *Follow a low-fat diet.* "A diet low in saturated fat aimed at about a daily intake of 20 percent fat, coupled with a restricted carbohydrate intake to reduce insulin production, should be the cornerstone of any diet for prostate and heart health," explains Dr. Strum.
- *Limit calories.* Caloric restriction to 500 calories per meal, adjusted to the individual's level of activity and body mass, says Dr. Strum, is another major step to reduce prostate cancer growth.
- *Eat more tomato-based foods.* Tomatoes anyone? Dr. Strum knows that eating tomatoes and tomato sauce is good for a healthy prostate because they contain lycopene (an antioxidant-rich red carotenoid pigment).

  It is reported by the National Cancer Institute that the higher the intake and blood levels of lycopene, the lower the risk of prostate cancer.
- *Try vitamins like selenium and vitamin E.* Supplements containing the disease-fighting antioxidants selenium and vitamin E may help to lower the risk of developing cancer of the prostate gland. This should begin at age 25 and become a lifelong practice.

RESEARCH IN A NUTSHELL

According to a study published in the *Journal of the National Cancer Institute*, in a double-blind trial that involved 29,133 smokers, those who were given 50 milligrams of synthetic vitamin E daily for five to eight years showed a 32 percent reduction in prostate cancer and a 41 percent drop in prostate cancer deaths. (Heinonen OP, Albanes P, Virtamo J, et al. "Prostate cancer and supplementation with alpha-tocopherol and beta-carotene: incidence and mortality in a controlled trial." *Journal of the National Cancer Institute*, 1998; 90:440–446)

MALE MENOPAUSE

Surprise! According to Dr. Strum, male menopause is as common as female menopause; it's just not discussed. "Male menopause is the most understated aspect of aging in our society. Male menopause or 'andropause' is supposedly more subtle than female menopause. Some deny its existence," he explains.

But the fact is, it does indeed exist, says Dr. Strum. "As a medical oncologist, focused for years only on the diagnosis and treatment of prostate cancer, it is clear to me that the deprivation of male hormone, testosterone, abruptly pushes men into full-blown andropause with exaggerated and accelerated signs and symptoms that yield clear but painful clues."

So what are the telltale signs of male menopause, anyhow? Dr. Strum told me that he has experienced many of these symptoms in himself. And since he's been there, done that, he candidly tells it like it is:

- Men see hair thinning from the tops of their heads only to crop up and grow furiously on their ears and in their nose.
- Nails are more brittle and skin loses its elasticity.
- Cognitive changes become apparent as you forget names of movie stars or sports figures or just can't remember the name of the person you bumped into on the street.

- Your erections no longer support a beach towel as they did in yesteryears and now can barely manage a regular bath towel.
- Your urine stream is not like that of the young guy in his teens or twenties; you can still be standing at a public urinal while two younger guys have come and gone.
- To add insult to injury, you have lost some of that muscle tone, and the midline bulge is creeping up on you.
- You notice a little breast enlargement as testosterone levels drop and the testosterone/estrogen ratio shifts in favor of estrogen.

What can be done to prevent or treat this mixed bag of woes? After you read Dr. Strum's recommendations, I urge you to go directly to Chapter 33, "Weight Loss," and on to Chapter 35, "Anti-Aging," for more helpful advice.

Meanwhile, get a baseline endocrine profile that tells you exactly what the status of your hormonal levels are. "I want to encourage men at the age of 25 to initiate such a baseline and to repeat such testing at five-year intervals. We need to start to think of our body in the way we think about car maintenance. If our car's carburetor was too rich in fuel and not in oxygen we would ask the mechanic to make the proper adjustment. We are not doing that as we age," says Dr. Strum. And let's face it, as the hormonal axis begins to falter we need to maintain balance.

"If men decide upon hormone replacement using DHEA, androstenedione, or testosterone patches or gel, they need someone to medically supervise blood levels of these biologic markers and adjust the doses for an individual's needs," warns Dr. Stephen Strum. "Moreover, it is advisable for patients wanting to preserve their hormonal balance to work with physicians who are knowledgeable in this arena."

THE DOC'S MALE MENOPAUSE REMEDY LIST

Here are some supplements and lifestyle measures that Dr. Strum recommends to his patients.

Male-Menopause Symptoms	Remedies	What They Do
Bone changes	Exercise, calcium, multi-mineral supplements, bi-phosphonates	Prevents bone loss
Cognitive dysfunction	Ginkgo biloba	Helps stimulate memory
Genitalia changes	Frequent sexual activity, Viagra	Maintains libido
Emotional changes	Hormone replacement therapy, meditation, support groups	Prevents anxiety, stress, loneliness
Nail changes	Gelatin, calcium, and magnesium supplements	Strengthens nails
Skin changes	Alpha hydroxy acid topical ointment	Exfoliates skin's surface, leaving fresher layers
Prostate cancer	Vitamin E, selenium supplements	Helps combat cancer
Skeletal muscle loss	Muscle-building exercises L-carnitine (amino acid supplement), restricted carbohydrate diet	Supports muscle mass

Urine flow changes	Saw palmetto combined with pygeum africanum and stinging nettle	Maintains a healthy pros- tate

Safety Smarts: Selenium: It can be harmful in high doses. Do not take more than 600 mcg daily. Saw palmetto: Do not use until you see a doctor first. If you have an enlarged prostate it is important to exclude prostate cancer before using saw palmetto. Viagra: Do not take Viagra if you are taking ni- trates or nitroglycerin-containing medicines. Do talk with your doctor be- fore using this prescribed drug.

DOC'S RX TO HEAL YOURSELF

- Eat a low-fat, moderate-calorie diet.
- Eat more tomato-based foods to prevent prostate cancer.
- Try antioxidants selenium and vitamin E.
- Get a baseline test to evaluate your hormone levels, and con- sult with your doctor about hormonal balance if need be.
- Take calcium supplements to aid in preventing bone loss.
- Don't forget saw palmetto for BPH and prostate cancer pre- vention or treatment.
- Supplements helpful for keeping a strong memory include ginkgo biloba.
- Use it or lose it—from exercise to sex—to improve your sense of well-being.

BIO

Stephen Strum, M.D., attended the University of Chicago School of Medicine. He is an oncologist and currently the medical direc- tor of the Prostate Cancer Research Institute (PCRI), a nonprofit organization in Los Angeles after 30 years in private practice in southern California. At 58, he is married with two children and resides in Los Angeles. The PCRI web site is at www.prostate-cancer.org.

29

Prostate Cancer

Dr. Magaziner's Secondhand Story

ALLAN MAGAZINER, D.O.

About seven years ago, at age 70, Dr. Allan Magaziner's father was diagnosed with prostate cancer. And his son, a preventive health care doctor, candidly told me how he helped his father to fight the battle and regain his health.

While he didn't have any symptoms, the doctor's father was getting an annual checkup. "He was found to have an elevated prostate-specific antigen on a routine blood test. If it's elevated it can mean many things. One, it can mean that there is an inflammation of the prostate gland. Usually what they'll do if it's high (after rechecking it) is do a prostate biopsy." After a wait-and-see approach they did exactly that in his father's case.

"We were concerned. I wasn't alarmed because it is a very common problem as men get over the age 60 or 70," explains Dr. Magaziner, who knows that if prostate cancer is caught early, before it spreads, it is treatable. "Fortunately in his case it had not metastasized. We did do a bone scan and it did not appear to have spread into the bone."

So how did they treat it? "Initially I started him on nutrients and supplements. But he also received hormonal therapy. A conventional urologist gave him injections to shut off the production of testosterone. But he ran into so much depression from these injections of hormones (because they shut off his testosterone). His whole zest for life was taken away from him and he became extremely depressed. He could hardly get off the couch for about three months. And this was a guy that was working full-time."

Dr. Magaziner continues, "First of all, I told him to get off the shots. Then, I put him on a group of nutrients as well." (See "The Doc's Supplement List" on page 227.) Meanwhile, Dr. Magaziner's father is doing well clinically. And Dr. Magaziner believes that his dad's story is something men need to know about. "He did not receive any chemotherapy, radiation, or surgery," he points out. "The only thing he received was the hormone injections."

As a preventive measure, Dr. Magaziner, who believes he is at higher risk because his father had prostate cancer, eats a lot of tomatoes and takes supplemental selenium and vitamin E, which may help him to lower his risk of developing the disease. He also takes saw palmetto, which has enjoyed a long history of being used to relieve male urinary discomfort caused by an enlarged prostate. According to the July/August 2000 issue of *Energy Times,* this herb (*Serenoa repens*) has been employed for several hundred years by Native Americans. Its berries were brewed into a tea and drunk for urinary and sexual problems. The beneficial components of the saw palmetto are found in fat-soluble extracts, which contain fatty acids, natural substances called plant sterols and flavonoids. And it's these extracts that are believed to be effective in reducing BPH symptoms.

PHYSICAL CHECKUP

The good news is that prostate cancer—the most prevalent cancer in men—is almost always curable when caught early. A digital rectal exam detects it; a blood test called prostate-specific antigen (PSA) can confirm the diagnosis.

THE DOC'S SUPPLEMENT LIST

The following supplements are what Dr. Magaziner prescribed to his father as treatment for prostate cancer.

Supplement	What It Does
Lycopene	A phytonutrient that may increase the lifespan of people who already have cancer
Selenium and vitamin E	Both of these antioxidants can help provide protection against cancer

DOC'S RX TO HEAL YOURSELF

- Get a regular PSA test to detect prostate cancer early on.
- Include antioxidant supplements vitamin E, selenium, and lycopene to help maintain a healthy prostate.

BIO

Allan Magaziner, D.O., at 44, is a practicing physician and one of the nation's authorities on nutritional, preventive, and environmental medicine. He is a graduate of Chicago College of Osteopathic Medicine in Chicago, Illinois. He is the author of *Achieving Optimal Health* and *The Complete Idiot's Guide to Living Longer and Healthier* (Alpha Books) and founder and director of the Magaziner Medical Center in Cherry Hill, New Jersey.

PART VIII

Mind, Body, and Spirit

Ever wish you knew how to feel good from head to toe? If the answer is a resounding "yes!" you might want to open your mind to this final section, Part VIII, "Mind, Body, and Spirit." I know it sounds strange—I was skeptical myself. But I decided to give it a try.

I spoke to some of our nation's top doctors and gave myself a homework assignment: tune into my mind and body and try to disconnect from the exterior world. I hate homework assignments, so I just let it slip by—until I was having a particularly bad day. I took a walk in the middle of my workday. I escaped to the lake and walked on the shore for a while. Then I plopped my body on the sand, stretched out, and stared at the boats. Both my body and my mind were at peace. It was such a comfort. I was in heaven.

I was shocked! Was this really happening? Was it just a coincidence?

The doctors in this section, and many of the people they have helped to make a connection with their body and mind, say it's no coincidence. By using diet, supplement, and lifestyle strategies, as I did, you too can get that body and mind fix—a place we can all find.

Drs. Diana Bihova and Kahlil Khatri provide tips for your

skin that can boost your body and spirit. Both an ophthalmologist, Robert Abel Jr., M.D., and an optometrist, Charles Krall, O.D., discuss how to maintain good eyesight at any age. And Dr. Victor Zeines and other tooth-savvy dentists will tell you how to keep your teeth healthy at any age.

How to pare pounds is a big problem for people of all ages. Drs. Jan McBarron and Julian Whitaker will tell you how to lose weight for good. Plus, Dr. John P. Foreyt shows you how to practice his motto: "Living without dieting. It's a new lifestyle," he says.

Pain management through eating the right foods? You bet, according to Neal Barnard, M.D. And anti-aging secrets are provided by Dr. Arnold Fox and other doctors who have found their own fountain of youth.

While you're feeling good, tips on fueling the libido will help you maintain sexual health at any age. Drs. Cynthia Watson and Steven Lamm share their inside expertise.

You can keep healthy by being on top of environmental toxins, and Drs. Elson Haas, Flemming Fuller Royal, and other doctors will tell you just how to keep your body and mind clear of unwanted pollution.

Meanwhile, understanding the link between spirituality and health will feed your soul. And Dr. Dean Edell, who has dished out health advice to the nation, talks about *his* personal stay-healthy routine.

To round out *Doctors' Orders: What 101 Doctors Do to Stay Healthy*, I'm bringing you words of wisdom from Drs. Richard Huemer and Sarah Brewer. Both doctors and a few others provide you with insight to the future to keep you and your loved ones healthy for generations to come. Here's to your good health—for maintaining a healthy body, mind, and soul.

30

Skin Problems

HEALTHY SKIN BY DR. BIHOVA

DIANA BIHOVA, M.D.

64

To achieve younger-looking and healthier skin easily, whether you're 20 years old or 50 years old plus, here's exactly what your skin needs—at every age, according to dermatologist Dr. Diana Bihova.

In Your Twenties

- *Primary skin problem.* Acne, also known as pimples, consists of inflamed and painful swellings (sometimes pus-filled) due to oily secretions from the skin's sabacous glands clogging hair follicles. Blame these red spots, often found on the face, back, or shoulders, on hormones or bacteria.
- *Diet.* Foods that are rich in iodine (seafood, kelp) can trigger an acne flare-up. Also, drinking milk more three times a day can make a person who has a tendency to break out be more likely to develop acne lesions.

   Zinc, an antioxidant trace mineral, may reduce acne, regulate oil glands, and clear problem skin. Good food sources include fish, nuts, beans, and grains. However, supplements alone cannot prevent acne.

Vitamin A, a protective antioxidant, is perhaps the most valuable skin nutrient to help prevent acne. Some good food sources are carrots, cantaloupes, apricots, and sweet potatoes.

- *Lifestyle.* If you can design a stress-free environment, you can control acne breakouts. While exercise can destress you, sweaty workouts can also trigger acne flare-ups. Rather than exercise, Dr. Bihova feeds her head and goes to the theater to chill out, which helps to keep her face clear.

In Your Thirties

- *Primary skin problem.* Rosacea looks like acne, sort of. It is a flushing or redness on the cheeks or nose that can sting or burn.
- *Diet.* Rosacea is more common in mature skin—over 30—and in fair-skinned people. Drinking hot coffee or tea can make rosacea flare up. While a glass of white wine can be relaxing, red wine can trigger rosacea. "I have a glass of white wine in the evening to unwind. It's good for your heart, your psyche, and your skin," says Dr. Bihova.

  Eating foods that contain tyramine, a substance that can dilate blood vessels, can contribute to rosacea. She tells her patients to avoid red wine, vinegar, tomatoes, spinach, beans, avocados, and raisins.
- *Lifestyle.* Like acne, exercise can trigger rosacea. However, if you change activities from sweat-inducing stationary bicycle riding to swimming this can be helpful, according to Dr. Bihova. Heat from exercise and sunlight can trigger rosacea. So switch your exercise routine if need be and shun the sun.

In Your Forties

- *Primary skin problem.* Dry skin, marked by flakiness and tightness, is due to the loss of moisture accompanying the loss of estrogen.
- *Diet.* Skin foods packed with protective antioxidants A and

E can help slow down loss of moisture associated with dry skin. Also, vitamin E can be applied directly to the skin via lotions and creams, as it is a highly moisturizing oil. Food sources of vitamin E include wheat germ, almonds, sunflower seeds, and legumes.

- *Lifestyle.* Dry spots, due to slower oil production, can be remedied. Fruit acids, also known as alpha hydroxy acids (AHAs), come to the rescue for dry skin, says Dr. Bihova. These natural substances are derived from fruit and milk products and work by chemically exfoliating the skin's surface, leaving a fresher layer exposed. AHAs may help reduce the appearance of noticeable lines, crow's feet, and fine wrinkles often linked with dry skin.

In Your Fifties

- *Primary skin problem.* Wrinkles—fine lines, deep lines, and crow's feet—result from sun damage, daily tension, and stress. The underlying cause is the loss of collagen, which gives skin its elasticity and firmness.
- *Diet.* The fact is, you don't have to be 60 to have wrinkles. "I see women in their thirties who already have quite a lot. "You have to have a healthy diet—vitamins, minerals, fruits, and vegetables can all help you have younger-looking skin," says Dr. Bihova.

  Vitamin C is known for slowing the breakdown of collagen, which means it works to keep skin elastic and supple. Some excellent sources of vitamin C are fruits such as cantaloupes, grapefruits, oranges, and strawberries.

  A combination of antioxidants A, C, and E can help slow down loss of elasticity and moisture associated with aging. "Aging has to do with free radical oxidation, which means that the waste products affect our skin on a cellular level when exposed to waste products such as skin-damaging sunlight and smoke," explains Dr. Bihova. It will help to take protective antioxidant supplements to ensure that you are getting an adequate amount daily.

- *Lifestyle.* Sun and genes play a role. Also, the way you use your facial muscles (laughing or frowning) can affect the skin and cause fine lines and wrinkles. However, these days we have Botox®, which simply relaxes the muscles. Botox® is a safe bacterial toxin that is injected into the skin, explains Dr. Bihova, who provides it for her patients.

The bottom line for women (and men) is that the antidote for healthy skin at any age requires eating a well-balanced diet and being sun-wise to prevent premature wrinkles and skin cancer.

THE DOC'S SUPPLEMENT LIST

Dr. Bihova recommends these supplements combined with lifestyle changes to get healthier and younger-looking skin at any age.

Supplement	What It Does
Vitamin A	This antioxidant may help provide a blemish-free complexion and slow down the elasticity and moisture loss linked with aging
Vitamin C	This antioxidant slows down the breakdown of collagen, which can work to keep skin elastic and supple
Vitamin E	This antioxidant may provide protection from ultraviolet light, reducing the appearance of fine lines and wrinkles
Zinc	This mineral may help to prevent acne, regulate oil glands, and clear problem skin

Safety Smarts: If you take too much vitamin C, it can cause gastrointestinal problems.

DR. KAHTRI'S SKIN SAVERS FOR MEN

KAHLIL KHATRI

The bare fact is, women seem to age in the face faster than men do. However, men do get wrinkles and "character lines," too.

Ever wonder what male dermatologists do to protect their own skin? Here are eight skin savers from dermatologist Dr. Kahlil Khatri, who provides his personal day-to-day strategies to avoid getting that sun-damaged "lizard" look.

1. Avoid sun exposure. Ultraviolet light (UV) rays can cause premature aging and skin cancer. Sunscreen 15 SPF (sun protection factor) for daily use is fine. However, if you are exposed to water, snow, or high altitudes Dr. Khatri advises you to use SPF 30 for ultimate protection. Skin experts claim the sun accounts for up to 90 percent of aging—wrinkles, blotches, liver spots, and leathery skin.

2. Avoid nicotine. Smoking can also cause aging skin around the mouth and eyes. Think fine lines above the upper lip and crow's feet. We know that if we compare smokers to nonsmokers, the smokers have more wrinkles than their nonsmoking counterparts.

3. Wear UV-protective eyeglasses. When you're outdoors, wear UV sunglasses for two reasons. When there is bright light you will squint, and that will cause lines on your forehead and around your eyes. The UV rays in sunlight can also cause cataracts and macular degeneration.

4. Take warm, quick showers. Do not take a long, hot shower. It can dry your skin. Use lukewarm water instead.

5. Eat right. The saying "You are what you eat" certainly can apply to skin, says Dr. Khatri. Usually, people who eat junk food have other bad habits such as drinking and smoking, which all can age the skin, whereas those who eat nutrient-dense diets are more prone to avoid unhealthy habits.

6. Exercise. Getting a move on—such as walking outdoors or on the indoor treadmill—can increase blood flow, which can give you that healthy glow.

7. Moisturize please. Right after a shower, don't rub your skin with a towel—just pat dry, and at that point you want to put on a moisturizer. It's not feminine, and it can keep your skin from cracking and drying. Try using chamomile lotion daily, because chamomile, which is a medicinal plant, can help prevent skin damage from sunburn and windburn.

8. Get mole smarts. Consult with your doctor if you see these changes in moles on your body: if it's asymmetrical; if borders are irregular or jagged; if it's multicolored; if the diameter is bigger than an eraser on a pencil head.

Docs' Rx to Heal Yourself

- Take protective antioxidant supplements A, C, E, and zinc for healthy and younger-looking skin.
- Be sun wise—protect your skin and eyes from UV rays.
- Forget smoking.
- Eat a healthful and balanced diet to feed your skin.
- Exercise regularly to promote blood circulation.
- Moisturize your skin to keep it supple.
- If you have any changes in moles, consult with your doctor.

Bios

Diana Bihova, M.D., is a 52-year-old board-certified dermatologist and has a private practice in New York City. She received her M.D. in the former Soviet Union. She is the author of *Beauty from the Inside Out* (Rawson Associates).

Kahlil Khatri, M.D., is a dermatologist and cosmetic laser surgeon. He is medical director of the Skin and Laser Surgery Center of New England, Cambridge, Massachusetts, and Nashua, New Hampshire. He attended Sindh Medical College in Karachi, Pakistan. At 44 he is married, has two children, and resides in Lexington, Massachusetts. Web site: www.skinlaseronline.com.

31

Eye Problems

FOCUSING BETTER WITH DR. ABEL'S VISION

ROBERT ABEL JR., M.D.

The first time I paid attention to my eyes was in graduate school. With all the studying I was doing, my eyes, were very red and burned a lot. I went to an ophthalmologist who said I had dry eye—a common problem. But it was a painful one to me.

As an ophthalmologist, Dr. Robert Abel is all too familiar with common problems like dry eye. And he also knows that sunlight, lifestyle, stress, and inadequate nutrition can wreak havoc on eye health. Here's Dr. Abel's treatment for himself and his patients.

Dry Eye. This is the number-one eye problem—having a deficient tear cell. We are a dehydrated society; we're not drinking enough water. You can also get dry eye from staring at a computer screen. When you don't blink and the eye dries out, the body dilates the blood vessels trying to leak fluids out to moisten the eye. In colder climates, indoor heat without humidity dehydrates the eye.

Rx. Drink filtered water. Remember to blink. Use a glare screen on your computer. Also, certain medications can be culprits that cause dryness of the eyes such as blood pressure medications, diuretics, and antihistamines. If possible, use natural remedies under the guidance of your health-care provider. Use a humidifier in a cold, dry climate.

Red Eye. Infections that can be caused by viruses or bacteria can end up as "red eye," also known as conjunctivitis. You can get it from touching a foreign object (such as money) and rubbing your eye or just being irritated from the swimming pool.

Rx. Don't rub your eyes. But note that red eye can also be due to an internal eye disease (such as acute glaucoma) as well as an external conjunctivitis. If you do not improve within a couple of days or if your vision should diminish, you should see an eye doctor. If you wear contact lenses, any red eye should be seen by a specialist because you could have a rapidly occurring corneal ulcer.

Cataracts. Cataracts are caused by a clouding of the proteins in the lens of the eye. The result: gradual blurred vision—usually more so at a distance than close up—for reading. "It's the number-one cause of blindness around the world," says Dr. Abel. Cataracts can be linked to age, sunlight, smoking, and poor nutrition.

"The concept here," explains Dr. Abel, "is that we breathe oxygen, which causes oxidation. The combination of the toxic short wavelength of light in conjunction with oxygen breaks down the crystalline proteins in the lens. The lens has antioxidants—vitamin C and glutathione—that diminish with age."

Rx. Wear sunglasses and take appropriate antioxidants including vitamin E.

Glaucoma. Glaucoma is "a group of conditions that feature optic nerve atrophy based on elevated pressure, decreased circulation, or decreased nerve protection. It can lead to blindness—an age-related problem," says Dr. Abel. "Glaucoma is a disease of emotional stress of the body. One of the major factors in glaucoma is low blood pressure at night. That means you have poor circulation to your head and your eyes."

Rx. "I recommend all glaucoma people to be on magnesium [good for circulation] at bedtime or ginkgo biloba, which is an herb that improves circulation," says Dr. Abel.

In addition, "Anything that relaxes you will improve circulation to the eye," says Dr. Abel. Also, "Exercise lowers eye pressure. Regular walking is as good as any one eyedrop. Deep breathing lowers eye pressure and improves circulation to the back of the eye. And if you can go even further and meditate 10 to 30 minutes a day, that may be the best way to solve your own glaucoma. It confirms the fact that it is a disease of stress."

Macular Degeneration. The macula is the middle area of the retina, which lets you see detail. Macular degeneration is "starvation of the retina [the retina becomes damaged]. It's the number-one cause of age-related blindness in developed countries. In America we have up to 20 million with macular degeneration, with the promise of an even greater number with increased longevity and decreased nutrition," says Dr. Abel.

Rx. "Again, our antioxidant friends come in. The low antioxidant level, chronic sun exposure, and saturated fat—these things have been studied. Fish eaters have less macular degeneration. Deep cold-water fish (salmon, tuna, cod, mackerel, and sardines).

"Lutein is one of the biggest items because it has been so well studied," says Dr. Abel. Lutein is a carotenoid (an antioxidant nutrient that improves eye health) found in spinach, kale, collard greens, rhubarb, and a lot of the yellow vegetables, even corn. Consuming lutein will not only increase your blood level and increase your macular pigment level, but it can help aid in the fight against macular degeneration.

THE DOC'S SUPPLEMENT LIST

These are some of the vitamins that Dr. Abel takes each day to care for his eyes.

Supplement	What It Does
Vitamin A	This fat-soluble antioxidant vitamin protects membranes against free radicals
Vitamin C	Antioxidant protects the lens from free radical damage, reducing the development of cataracts
Vitamin E	Antioxidant prevents free radicals from damaging the lens of the eye
Glutathione (made up of amino acids: cysteine, glutamic acid, and glycine)	An antioxidant that protects against free radicals and protects the eye from aging; may reduce risk of macular degeneration

Safety Smarts: Vitamin A: It can be toxic in large amounts (more than 10,000 IU) since it is stored in the liver. Vitamin C: If you take too much, it can cause gastrointestinal problems.

DR. KRALL'S ANTI-MACULAR DEGENERATION DIET

CHARLES KRALL, O.D.

What is macular degeneration? Just ask Dr. Charles Krall, an optometrist; he'll tell you. The bad news is, this condition is a chronic, progressive disease and the leading cause of blindness in adults over the age of 50. It happens when the tissue in the macula-the point in the retina that is responsible for central vision—deteriorates. The good news: Macular degeneration doesn't affect side vision, and usually doesn't cause 100 percent blindness. However, the loss of central vision—which you use for reading and driving—can impair your lifestyle.

Among the risk factors for macular degeneration according to Dr. Krall are the following:

- *Age.* Macular degeneration affects primarliy Caucasians who are age 65 or older.
- *Genes.* Heredity can play a role in developing this condition.
- *Sunlight.* Long-term exposure to shortwave ultraviolet light can cause damage to the retina.
- *Environmental pollution.* Cigarette smoke especially increases your risk.
- *Skin color.* Especially at risk are fair-skinned people with lighter-colored eyes, partly because they have less pigmentation in their eye. Sunlight is a factor that causes damage in the eye.
- *Blood pressure.* High blood pressure affects the circulation in the eye.
- *Diet.* People who maintain inadequate levels of antioxidant vitamins such as A, C, and E and selenium are at high risk.

Dr. Krall knows that evidence suggests that antioxidants can help protect against macular degeneration. After all, the culprit in this disease process is the production of free radicals. These free radicals are produced in the body through sunlight, radiation, and air pollution and are produced by each cell as it oxidizes or burns food into energy.

The body's protective system to scavenge these free radicals and terminate these chain reactions are vitamins, minerals, and enzymes. These defense nutrients are called antioxidants or free radical scavengers. The primary antioxidants are called the "Four Aces": vitamins A, C, and E and the mineral selenium.

Foods that are rich in the Four Aces are listed below. The

foods are listed top to bottom with the richest source at top. To ensure an adequate amount of these essential elements you may wish to take additional supplements.

Vitamin A	*Vitamin C*	*Vitamin E*	*Selenium*
RDA 5,000 IU	45 mg	15 IU	50–200 mg
Liver	Red peppers	Wheat germ oil	Shrimp
Red peppers	Chives	Hazelnuts	Smelt
Carrots	Guava	Almonds	Lobster
Crab	Parsley	Soybean oil	Scallops
Kale	Kale	Corn oil	Oysters
Sweet potatoes	Turnip greens	Peanuts	Beef liver
Parsley	Green peppers	Herring	Cod
Spinach	Collards	Cucumbers	Round steak
Collards	Broccoli	Kale	Flatfish
Turnip greens	Brussels sprouts	Mackerel	Brazil nuts
Swiss chard	Watercress	Beef liver	Lamb chops
Beet greens	Cauliflower	Safflower oil	Brown rice
Winter squash	Kiwi	Sesame oil	Whole-wheat products
Broccoli	Lemons	Turnip greens	Ground beef
Mango	Strawberries	Peanut oil	White rice
Green onions	Papayas	Whole-wheat bread	Clams
Cantaloupe	Oranges	Green peas	Bran
Papaya	Grapefruit	Brown rice	Chicken breast
Eggs	Cantaloupe	Asparagus	Cottage cheese

(Source: Krall Optometric Clinic)

PHYSICAL CHECKUP

Have an ophthalmologist or optometrist check your eyes every year or two. Some eye diseases don't have obvious early symptoms.

DOC'S RX TO HEALING YOURSELF

- Use lifestyle preventive measures such as wearing UV sunglasses, using a computer glare screen, and avoiding prolonged sunlight and cigarette exposure to protect your eyes.
- Include ginkgo biloba in your diet to prevent cataracts.
- Antioxidants A, C, E, and selenium from foods and supplements can help slow cataract growth and prevent macular degeneration.
- Getting a regular eye exam can help detect early signs of cataracts, glaucoma, and macular degeneration. If you notice any changes in your vision, consult with your eye doctor immediately.

BIOS

Robert Abel Jr., M.D., is an ophthalmologist who lives in Wilmington, Delaware. He is the author of *The Eye Care Revolution* (Kensington). At 57, he is married and has one son.

Charles Krall, O.D., a 67-year-old optometrist, received his O.D. at the Illinois Eye Institute in Chicago, Illinois. He currently has a practice, the Krall Optometric Clinic in Mitchell, South Dakota, where he lives. He is married and has six children.

32

Oral Problems

Dr. Zeines's Healthy Mouth Program

VICTOR ZEINES, D.D.S.

As a child I went to the dentist, and as a teenager I went to the orthodontist. Both experiences were unpleasant. These days, however, dentistry is more modern and less painful. What's more, we have more choices.

In his book *Healthy Mouth, Healthy Body* (Kensington), Dr. Victor Zeines, a classically trained dentist who began holistic therapy three decades ago, explains how "natural dentistry" can benefit the total body.

- *Amalgam fillings.* Holistic dentists, such as Dr. Zeines, stay clear of using silver amalgam fillings (a type of cavity filling of which half is mercury, a toxic metal), because they believe that eating and drinking can cause mercury to leak into the body.

  "Literally thousands of people have told me that when they have had mercury amalgam fillings removed, they sleep better or their memory has been improved. If you think about that for a minute," he told me, "what they're saying is that somehow the central nervous system was not functioning properly with the metal fillings in the mouth. Just getting them out seems to change things," says Dr. Zeines.

- *Root canals.* "When you have a root canal, picture a sponge with a billion little holes in it. Make one big hole in the middle of the sponge—that's the hole that gets filled when you do a root canal. All these other little holes are still there and they're filled with bacteria, so the tooth is still putting toxins into your body from all those other bacteria," explains Dr. Zeines. But today, "There are alternative ways of doing a root canal, using more biocompatible materials," says Dr. Zeines. "Alternative compounds (such as calcium hydroxide) are more compatible to our bodies."

  In addition, says Dr. Zeines, "I have my patients build up their immune system as well if they're about to have a root canal." Normal daily supplementation can do this. (For supplementation recommendations, see Chapter 14.)

- *Gum disease.* According to Dr. Zeines, you can prevent gum disease, also known as gingivitis. "You've got to eat well," he says. "What do you know about bears? Bears don't go to the dentist too often and they don't floss a lot. And most bears don't have problems with their teeth." The key: a natural, healthful diet.

  "Flossing is great. Brushing is greater. It's important to do it. But if you have a really good cleansing diet, high in fresh vegetables and fiber, that in itself will actually cleanse your teeth," says Dr. Zeines. "But eating is not enough. You've got to start taking supplements."

  Another gum-healthy remedy is to use a healing herbal gum rinse, says Dr. Zeines. "In three days you'll see an improvement in your mouth and gums."

  Adds Dr. Zeines, "We rebuild smiles. It's good for a lot of people because it gets people to smile more. When you smile more you have a better immune system."

THE DOC'S SUPPLEMENT LIST

Here are two key vitamins that Dr. Zeines takes in supplement form and recommends to his patients to maintain healthy teeth and gums.

Nutrient	What It Does	Food Sources
Calcium	This mineral protects your bones and teeth (women with strong bones are more likely to keep their teeth than women who lose bone density to osteoporosis)	Low-fat yogurt, low-fat cheese, sardines and canned salmon (with the bones)
Vitamin C	This antioxidant keeps your gums healthy, helps gums that bleed after flossing	Citrus fruits, strawberries, green and red peppers, and broccoli

Safety Smarts: If you take too much vitamin C, it can result in gastrointestinal problems.

Dr. Cerceo Grills Fillings

CHRIS ALLEN CERCEO, D.D.S.

I asked my dentist, Dr. Chris Cerceo, whether mercury amalgam fillings (the silver fillings that you and I have for dental cavities) are safe. Is it really worth your time and money to face the drill and replace those fillings with a nontoxic ceramic composite material? Listen up, and decide for yourself. In his own words, Dr. Cerceo speaks out:

Dental amalgam has been in use for over 150 years as a dental restorative material, and has functioned well as a direct-placement, single-visit filling. It is easy to use and is relatively inexpensive, and the corrosion that takes place at the tooth interface helps seal the inside of the tooth, even if not placed perfectly. However, more tooth structure must be removed to retain it within the tooth than with the alternative composite resins. As such, it can weaken the tooth if used injudiciously.

Opponents of amalgam report that neurological and immune suppression illnesses can be linked to its use, as a result of mercury vaporization that occurs during the chewing cycle. It is well known that ingestion of mercury is cumulative in one's lifespan and tends to result in higher concentrations in organisms at the top of the food chain.

Though the harmful effects of mercury are unquestionable, the damaging effects from the quantity of mercury ingested by individuals with dental fillings remain arguable at this time. And except for isolated instances where individuals have gained relief from chronic illnesses after having dental amalgams removed, the claims have not been substantiated by scientific double-blind experimentation and are largely anecdotal.

For individuals who have documented reactions to nonprecious metals, alternative restorative materials such as porcelain (silicon), gold, and composite (silica within a resin matrix) are suggested. All have one or more advantages over dental amalgam, with porcelain and composite having the added advantage of blending with the natural color of the tooth. No known illnesses, other than a rouge contact dermatitis, have been attributed to these alternative restorative materials.

Though the American Dental Association condones the use of amalgam and recognizes its place in the dentist's armamentarium when necessary, the recommended disposal of excess amalgam leaves us in a quandary regarding its safety. After all, there are just two ways to dispose of dental amalgam. Have it picked up and disposed of by a licensed hazardous waste transport company, or just place it in your teeth.

Meanwhile, I personally still have a few amalgam fillings from yesteryear sitting in my molars, causing no apparent harm. Dr. Cerceo believes it's better to let well enough alone since I am not having any problems. And it's my choice, for now, to let them be.

DR. VELIGDAN'S ANTI-GRINDING RX

ROBERT VELIGDAN, D.M.D.

People who gnash their teeth at night—a condition called sleep bruxism—can end up with sore jaws, eroded and shifting teeth, and damaged gums and bone, says Dr. Robert Veligdan, who estimates that 20 to 40 percent of his patients may grind their teeth while they sleep at one time or another.

To help control tooth grinding and its problems, take the following steps, which Dr. Veligdan follows himself.

- *Limit sugar, caffeine, and alcohol use.* These can interfere with calcium absorption, which is important for muscle metabolism, says Dr. Veligdan. "While caffeine will increase muscle tension and make the body more tense, which will cause the jaw to clench down more, sugar stresses you like alcohol. All of these give you an agitated sleep. You don't sleep as well."
- *Try herbal teas before bedtime.* To help you sleep, try a cup of chamomile, skullcap, or passionflower tea, recommends Dr. Veligdan. "Anything that makes you calm will decrease grinding."
- *Learn some relaxation techniques.* When you are stressed out the cortisol levels in your body are increased, which causes increased tension. "We take it out in the mouth," says Dr. Veligdan. The solution: "I meditate for 15 minutes every day. It reduces the pressure of the grinding," he says, adding that smiling and laughter help to destress the body, too.
- *Get physical.* Exercise is good because it eliminates stress from the body. "But if you overexercise you'll start tensing.

If you lift weights, consider wearing a nightguard if you clench your teeth as you lift the weights," says Dr. Veligdan.
- *Consult with your dentist about tooth protection measures.* Further treatments such as a nightguard, which is a protective dental device, may help to protect your teeth.

THE DOC'S SUPPLEMENT LIST

Dr. Veligdan takes and recommends these vitamins and minerals to minimize nighttime grinding and its effects.

Supplement	What It Does
Vitamin B complex	B vitamins help to release stress
Vitamin C	This antioxidant reduces inflammation of the joints, muscles, and gums from clenching the teeth
Calcium citrate orotate	This mineral helps muscle metabolism and relaxes you
DL-phenylalanine	It's an amino acid that helps induce endorphins, the body's natural painkillers in the body
Manganese	To help ligaments to heal
Magnesium	This mineral helps muscle metabolism; it reduces the stress in the body
Omega-3 fatty acids	Fish oils act as an anti-inflammatory

Safety Smarts: Vitamin C: If you take too much, it can cause gastrointestinal problems. Omega-3 fatty acids: Don't take high doses of fish oil capsules if you are taking NSAIDs (nonsteroidal anti-inflammatory drugs). It may increase gastrointestinal ulcers and bleeding.

PRESERVING KIDS' BITE WITH DR. MITTELMAN

JEROME S. MITTELMAN, D.D.S.

Ever wonder why some kids' teeth are healthy and others' are not? Well, a lot of it has to do with good pre- and postnatal care.

That's right, what supplements Mom takes during her pregnancy and what supplements she gives to her child make a difference, according to Dr. Jerome S. Mittelman and Beverly Mittelman, coauthors of *Healthy Teeth for Children* (Kensington).

PHYSICAL CHECKUP

Get a dental checkup twice a year to preserve your pearly whites.

THE DOC'S SUPPLEMENT LIST

Here are some nutrients that are essential for kids' teeth, according to Dr. and Mrs. Mittelman. Some are for prenatal care and others are for after birth for the child. And note: "Children need vitamins after birth from day one," says Beverly Mittelman.

Supplement	What It Does
Calcium (pre- and postnatal)	This mineral is for healthy bones and teeth
Vitamin A (prenatal)	For normal formation of the child's teeth
Vitamin C (pre- and postnatal)	An antioxidant important in the formation of dentin (layer of the tooth under enamel)

Vitamin D (pre- and postnatal)	A vitamin for healthy bones and teeth
Vitamin E (after birth for the child)	Antioxidant for healthy gums
Folic acid (prenatal)	B vitamin to prevent cleft lip and cleft palate
Iron (after birth for the child)	A mineral that can prevent cavities
Protein (prenatal)	It will help prevent crooked teeth and cavities (get at least 80 grams daily)
Zinc	A mineral important to prevent cleft palate

Safety Smarts: Vitamin A: Don't exceed 10,000 IU of preformed vitamin A (not beta carotene). Vitamin C: If you take too much, it can cause gastrointestinal problems.

RESEARCH IN A NUTSHELL

More tea, fewer cavities—that's what Dr. Christine Wu, of the University of Illinois at Chicago, reported to the American Society for Microbiology at its 101st meeting in Orlando, Florida.

She said, "If sequenced properly between meals and normal hygiene, drinking black tea could reduce the number of cavities and [help] prevent periodontal disease." Her subjects rinsed for one minute ten times a day. Multiple rinsings were necessary to prevent the bacterial growth.

Chemicals in black tea, polyphenols, suppress the growth of cavity causing bacterial plaque and reduce acid productions level. (*The Holistic Dental Digest Plus* no. 132: July–August 2001.)

Doc's Rx to Heal Yourself

- Discuss amalgam filling removal with your dentist.
- Brush and floss daily to keep your teeth and gums healthy.
- Supplement a healthy diet with calcium to protect your teeth and bones and vitamin C to keep your gums healthy.
- To control nighttime grinding, limit your intake of sugar, caffeine, and alcohol.
- Consider taking anti-grinding supplements such as calcium citrate, vitamin B complex, C, manganese, magnesium, CoQ_{10}, Omega fatty acids, and DL-Phenylalanine.
- Remember pre- and postnatal care supplements—vitamins A, C, E, D, calcium, folic acid, iron, protein, and zinc—to help keep your kids' teeth healthy.

Bios

Chris Allen Cerceo, D.D.S., received his D.D.S. at the College of Physicians and Surgeons of the University of the Pacific in Stockton, California. He co-owns his South Lake Tahoe, California–based general dentistry practice, Tahoe Family Dentists, with his wife Jeanie F. Kaufman. He is a member of both the American Dental Association and the American Academy of Cosmetic Dentistry. At 48, he is married, has two children, and resides in South Lake Tahoe.

Jerome S. Mittelman, D.D.S., is a retired dentist. He received his D.D.S. degree from the University of Pennsylvania in Philadelphia, Pennsylvania. He resides in New York City, is 78, is married, and has one child. He is the publisher of *The Holistic Dental Digest Plus,* a bimonthly newsletter.

Robert Veligdan, D.M.D., is assistant clinical professor at Columbia University Dental School in New York City. He graduated from the University of Pittsburgh School of Dental Medicine in Pittsburgh, Pennsylvania. He is 52 and lives in New York City.

Victor Zeines, D.D.S., has been practicing holistic dentistry for 30 years. He received his D.D.S. at New York University in New York City. He is a member of the American Dental Association and practices in Woodstock, New York, and New York City. He is single.

33

Weight Problems

DR. MCBARRON'S MIRACLE DIET

JAN MCBARRON, M.D.

Obesity: the statistics are sobering. One in four adults are over-weight. But as unhealthy as this may seem, we're not powerless. We don't have to use willpower and turn to fad diets. There are healthy steps we can take to take it off—and keep it off. And one of the most important is to adopt a healthful nutrient-dense diet and an aerobic exercise plan that works for you.

To help you determine the best weight loss program, I consulted with weight loss specialist Jan McBarron, M.D. Here, she shares the basis for her own personal fat-fighting diet.

"If I could do it, anyone can." That's exactly what Dr. McBarron assures the patients who come to her with seemingly hopeless weight problems. And they believe her, she told me, because they know she's speaking from experience. More than ten years ago, Dr. McBarron dropped 70 pounds from her 5'10" frame—and kept the weight off.

For a decade, Dr. McBarron fought a battle with her weight. "I lost 50 pounds—five times!" she says. "I tried every diet you can name. I finally attained my dream of becoming a doctor, but

I was miserable because I weighed over 200 pounds! It was time to get off the roller coaster." The meal plan that helped her has helped more than ten thousand of her patients. The doctor's meal plan is based on these principles:

- *Eat heartily early in the day.* Consuming the bulk of your calories in the morning means you have more time to burn them off. Dr. McBarron tells her patients, "Eat like a king at breakfast, a queen at lunch, and a pauper at dinner."

  Also, fat-burning enzymes work harder in the morning. "Food eaten in the morning is burned off more quickly than food eaten at night," says Dr. McBarron.
- *Focus on complex carbohydrates.* A diet of 70 percent complex carbohydrates—vegetables, fruits, pasta, rice, bread, lentils, peas, beans—provides more energy than one full of protein-rich foods, so you'll burn more fat, says Dr. McBarron. "Complex carbohydrates also stimulate the production of serotonin, a brain chemical that can ease the stress that leads to overeating."
- *Keep protein intake moderate.* "I restrict meat to one serving a day," says Dr. McBarron. "Meat is high in fat and has no fiber, while bulky, fiber-rich carbs fill you up so you eat less."
- *Have small snacks throughout the day.* "Healthy snacks stave off hunger," explains Dr. McBarron. "They also help keep my blood sugar levels on even keel, which helps prevent binges."
- *Lower fat intake.* "Only 10 to 20 percent of your total calories should come from fat. That's only 1 to 2 grams of fat for every 100 calories," says Dr. McBarron. "Also, I drink at least eight 8-ounce glasses of water a day."
- *Get moderate exercise.* "Walking is an excellent aerobic, fat-burning exercise. And consistency, not intensity, is the key to successful weight loss," says Dr. McBarron. For best results, she walks 30 minutes at least five times a week.

THE DOC'S SUPPLEMENT LIST

Also an expert in nutrition, Dr. McBarron practices what she preaches and adds these dietary supplements and herbs to her daily diet:

Supplement	What It Does
Multivitamin-and-mineral supplement	It must contain the B vitamins, inositol, and PABA (a part of the vitamin B complex). "They are necessary for carbohydrate metabolism, to cut food cravings, and to keep the kidneys in good shape."
Calcium	"I take 1,000 milligrams with 300 milligrams of magnesium plus boron and silica, which aids calcium absorption."
Chromium picolinate	200 micrograms daily. "This mineral regulates blood sugar levels and keeps a lid on insulin, which is an appetite stimulant and fat-making hormone."
Metabolic enhancer	"It revs up my fat-burning engine and is a natural appetite suppressant. I take one a day."
Spirulina	"Pure plant protein and an excellent, nonstimulating appetite suppressant. The window of safety is huge. If I'm hungry and can't stop for a meal, I take five or six tablets with a glass of water. It cuts my hunger."

SECOND OPINION: DR. WHITAKER'S WEIGHT LOSS PLAN

JULIAN WHITAKER, M.D.

As a health and fitness writer, I used to write about weight loss for several magazines. I discovered that people who won the battle of the bulge didn't reap the reward of pound-paring success by following fad or crash diets and doing sit-ups 25 hours a day. In fact, strict diets that promise a big weight loss just trigger the "starve-and-binge mentality." This, in turn, leads to weight gain and even more unwanted pounds.

People nationwide want to lose weight for good. And that includes health-conscious doctors, such as Julian Whitaker, M.D. He candidly told me that he has had a problem with weight loss. "I currently am about 30 pounds overweight," he says and points out that he is 5'11" and weighs in at 232 pounds. "If I weigh between 200 and 215 then I'm going to be happy, because I have a lot of muscle, too. My body fat is 22 percent."

And these days, Dr. Whitaker is following his custom-tailored weight loss plan geared to fire up his metabolism. So far, in five weeks he has lost 11 pounds. "If you lose 2 pounds a week and stay on the diet for nine weeks you've lost [almost] 20 pounds," he points out.

The answer lies in metabolism. The basal metabolic rate—that is, the rate at which your body burns calories when it's at rest—determines how quickly you lose weight. When your metabolism is in higher gear, you burn more calories, making it easier to lose weight and keep it off.

Dr. Whitaker is following a diet and exercise plan that boosts his metabolism into a higher, calorie-burning gear. He's eating regularly, starting the day off with breakfast, revving up his engine with complex carbs such as fiber-rich vegetables, adding some protein to his plate, and getting a move on.

Aerobic activity, such as brisk walking or tennis, is key to burning fat and calories. Dr. Whitaker exercises twice a day playing a racket sport such as squash or tennis. Aim for 30 minutes of exercise daily (it takes at least 20 minutes to elevate your heart rate to a fat-burning level). And remember, drink eight 8-ounce glasses of water or green tea daily (Dr. Whitaker drinks twelve) to help your body operate more efficiently.

RESEARCH IN A NUTSHELL

Green tea extract is a healthy herbal supplement that is believed to boost metabolism. According to European researchers, green tea, like other fat-burning foods, has a thermogenic effect, meaning that it helps your body produce heat to burn calories.

"Studies show that taking green tea twice a day can help reduce the formation of excess fat cells and curb appetite," reports Nadine Taylor, M.S., R.D., in her book *Green Tea: The Natural Secret for a Healthier Life* (Kensington).

SAMPLE ONE-DAY METABOLISM-BOOSTING DIET PLAN

To steadily lose weight, Dr. Whitaker's low-fat weight loss regimen is 1,200 to 1,500 calories per day. He drinks filtered water throughout the day (twelve 8-ounce glasses) and green tea (which contains natural chemicals that encourage your body to burn fat faster). Dr. Whitaker also drinks 24 ounces of low-sodium V-8. "It has an exceptionally high level of potassium. It's got the juice of eight vegetables. It has 620 milligrams of potassium. Each can contains only 35 calories."

Before Breakfast: One cup of coffee (stimulates the burning of calories). Combination of energy-boosting supplements such as pyruvate and carnitine. "Then I go play tennis for 40 minutes and work up a sweat."

Breakfast: Protein drink with about 40 to 50 grams of protein. (Dr. Whitaker adds some glutamine and creatine powder to increase the muscle replenishment, and powdered multi-vitamins high in antioxidants.)

Lunch: Fish and a salad. "I selectively avoid bread." (Dr. Whitaker uses an oil-based and vinegar dressing or a good low-fat dressing if it's available.)

Snack: Health bar.

Dinner: Poultry such as chicken and a salad chock-full of to-matoes, onions, bell peppers, broccoli, and cauliflower.

THE DOC'S SUPPLEMENT LIST

Here are some of the fat-burning nutrients Dr. Whitaker takes to help him slim down.

Supplement	What It Does
Carnitine	An amino acid that boosts energy
Creatine	A protein that can enhance athletic performance and increase lean muscle mass
Glutamine	An amino acid that nourishes the cells that line your intestines
Green tea	An herbal extract that contains natural chemicals that can help your body burn fat faster
Protein powder	It is rich in amino acids, which helps to build muscle, which can help to burn fat
Pyruvate	A nutrient that may increase energy

Safety Smarts: Creatine can cause kidney problems.

WEIGHT LOSS SECRETS FROM DRS. FOREYT, GIANNETTO, SHINTANI, WURTMAN, AND BRUNER

There may not be one particular diet plan for everyone, but there definitely are certain eating strategies that will guarantee success for all. I went to the country's top doctors with special expertise in weight loss and asked them for the best ways to lose the weight they want—and keep it off. Here's what they had to say:

JOHN P. FOREYT, PH.D.

"People equate the word *diet* with deprivation. That's not a good motivator," says John P. Foreyt, Ph.D. "Willpower always fails under times of stress because physiology beats psychology. It might work for a little while, while you're highly motivated, but in the long run, you don't want to rely on willpower."

Instead, the doctor tries to follow a set of lifestyle skills so he can maintain his weight throughout life. "I try to jog every day. The only time I miss is when I'm out of town. That's my problem—traveling."

Worse, when the doctor is on the road he is faced with the temptation of restaurant food. "That's the problem I have. I suffer when I travel out of town because other people are serving my food so I give somebody else the right to feed me rather than feed myself. I try to eat healthily and sensibly but it certainly isn't as good as when I have control over my own eating," Dr. Foreyt explains.

When Dr. Foreyt returns from a business trip he takes charge and nips potential weight gain in the bud. "I cut back more than normal to account for my overeating on travel. I try to get a balance. But jogging 45 minutes every morning helps so I feel more in control of my life."

Plus, he takes the problem-solving approach. "First, I set goals. I look at the steps needed to achieve those goals. I draw up a plan—laying out my jogging clothes next to my bed and setting the alarm earlier. I don't have to rely on willpower," he says. "I just have to rely on a problem-solving set of plans."

LISA GIANNETTO, M.D.

Exercise is the ticket to Dr. Lisa Giannetto's health plan. "I'm a very small person, about 5'2" inches and 98 pounds. But I find that if I don't exercise, my mental health deteriorates," she told me.

Therefore, on a regular basis she runs (she just finished a marathon), uses an elliptical trainer (the machine that gives you a workout similar to running without the impact on your knees), as well as some biking. "I will do aerobics or a cardiovascular exercise five to six times a week taking one day off. I'll do strength training or flexibility exercise two to three days a week," she explains.

"I don't have a weight problem, but it makes me look better. I would look scrawny if I didn't do some weight training. It gives me energy," she points out. "My body fat percentage is very low." Also, because she is a small-boned person the doctor turns to weight-bearing and strength-training exercises in addition to getting adequate calcium to try to prevent bone loss.

Dr. Giannetto adds, "I also find that in many women over age 45, the body changes. We tend to accumulate (even though we're fit and thin) more fat and weight in our stomach. It's very important for perimenopausal women to exercise. I see women saying, 'I'm not doing anything differently yet I've gained 5 to 10 pounds and it's all in my middle.' I tell them, 'You really have to fight back.' And the key to that is strength training along with their aerobic exercise."

A bonus exercise benefit: "I have a strong family history of cardiovascular disease. My father has coronary disease; my brother actually had a bypass surgery in his late thirties. Now, while I have a normal cholesterol level, don't smoke, and am at a much lower risk—the importance of exercise in preventing disease is key."

TERRY SHINTANI, M.D.

Exactly how does Dr. Terry Shintani, M.D., maintain his weight and stay healthy at mid-life? The doctor told me he keeps the weight off by using the "mass index" table that he writes about in his Hawaii Diet books and used in his study published in the *Hawaii Medical Journal*. (Shintani TT, Beckham S, Brown AC, et al. "The Hawaii Diet (77 percent carbohydrate): ad libitum high carbohdyrate, low fat multi-cultural diet for the reduction of chronic disease factors: obesity, hypertension, hypercholesterolemia, and hyperglycemia." 2001; 60 (3):69–73)

While studying nutrition at Harvard, Dr. Shintani looked at the wide difference between the health and weight of people around the world. He began to realize that those on low-fat, high-carbohydrate ancient traditional diets remained slim and free of the diseases that plague us today, such as heart disease, cancer, stroke, and diabetes. Those who began eating high-fat animal products and highly refined foods became overweight and sick.

Even more startling was the fact that those who followed a traditional diet (78 percent carbohydrate) ate large amounts of carbohydrate and more food but weighed less than their counterparts in developed countries. The reason: One of the major differences in the types of food is the "mass index" (MI) of the food. Those who were slim—like Dr. Shintani—ate high-MI foods; those who became obese ate low-MI foods.

Among the high-mass foods are the following (the numbers are the mass index):

Zucchini, 32.1
Tomato, 27.3
Broccoli, 17.1
Carrots, 13
Oatmeal, 9.9
Apples, 9.4

Corn, 6.5
Garbanzo beans, 5.6
Sweet potatoes, 5.4

Nine low-mass foods are the following:

Potato chips, 2.3
Cheeseburger, 2.1
French fries, 1.7
Ham sandwich, 1.6
Danish pastry, 1.5
Cheddar cheese, 1.4
Doughnuts, 1.3
Sirloin, 1.2
Oil/lard, 0.6

"The MI food table shows how many pounds of a food are required to provide a day's worth of calories. Foods over 4.1 tend to make you lose weight; foods below can make you gain. The lower the number, the worse it is. It works like a charm. An average weight loss is 11.1 pounds in three weeks without calorie restriction. People ate more food but weighed less," explains Dr. Shintani, whose personal diet consists of high-mass foods, which keep him lean and healthy.

RESEARCH IN A NUTSHELL

According to a study based on these principles led by Terry Shintani, M.D., eating an old-fashioned native Hawaiian diet can slim you down. A group of urbanized, obese native Hawaiians revealed that eating a low-fat diet increases satiety and spontaneously reduces caloric intake without counting calories.

These Hawaiians, who had been eating a high-fat Western diet, were fed the traditional Hawaiian diet. All the foods were low in fat: taro (a starchy rootlike potato), poi (a mashed form of taro), sweet potato, yams, breadfruit, greens (fern shoots and leaves of taro), a variety of fruit, seaweed, fish, and chicken. All foods were served either raw or steamed in a manner that approximated ancient styles of cooking.

After three weeks on Dr. Shintani's program, there was a 41 percent spontaneous decrease in calorie intake; the average weight loss was 17 pounds; and blood pressure and cholesterol levels were significantly reduced. (Shintani TT, Hughes CK, Beckham SK, O'Connor HK. "Obesity and cardiovascular risk intervention through the ad libitum feeding of traditional Hawaiian Diet." *The American Journal of Clinical Nutrition.* 1991; 53:1647S–51S)

JUDITH WURTMAN, PH.D.

Dr. Judith Wurtman, coauthor of *The Serotonin Solution* (Fawcett Columbine), believes that if you eat the right foods you can break the pattern of emotional eating for good. And to stay a svelte 120 pounds at 5'5" she does just that.

To stay lean and feel calm Dr. Wurtman turns to carbos. "Carbohydrate foods will when eaten on a relatively empty stomach increase the production of a chemical in your brain called serotonin. Serotonin has two important functions for weight loss and emotional well-being. One, it regulates your mood and when it's made in sufficient quantity will decrease feelings of depression, anger, or restlessness and make you feel tranquil," she explains. "The second thing that it will do is increase feelings of fullness, so one feels better and is at the same time less hungry."

So when Dr. Wurtman feels stressed out (whether it's at work due to a paper rejected for publication or a doggie accident at home), rather than overeat, she turns to carbs for comfort.

She will grab three-quarters of a cup of Wheat Chex cereal without milk or half of a toasted pita bread. "If I really feel like having something sweet I might have a couple of fig newtons. Or if I feel that need to eat something even more substantial I might microwave a small potato," she says. And by combining exercise with her stress-breaker foods Dr. Wurtman stays cool and calm and maintains her weight.

DENISE BRUNER, M.D.

Surprise! Carbs aren't the weight loss secret for everyone, according to weight loss specialist Dr. Denise Bruner. "One of the things I learned in my residency was that I was sensitive to carbohydrates. I couldn't figure out why I had gained about 40 pounds. I was always hungry. Then I finally looked at things and figured out that I was eating bagels, toast, English muffins, and orange juice with coffee and a little sugar. And I was starving all day," she told me.

"So I experimented with a breakfast of cottage cheese and fresh fruit. I also tried three hard-boiled egg whites, one yolk, and fruit. That would keep me full most of the day. It was amazing what a difference that made. Personally I know that if you're doing that (and also drinking at least 64 ounces of water a day) you are really satisfied. I watched my hunger level go down. Then I was able to control the food and lose weight."

The principle is simple: It takes more energy to convert protein into fuel than it does to convert carbohydrates. Therefore, "your body is forced to burn its stored fat to make the protein in your diet into a useful source of energy," concludes Dr. Bruner. This results in weight loss since protein is also digested slowly, so it helps suppress your appetite and provide long-lasting satisfaction.

DOCS' RX TO HEAL YOURSELF

- Eat healthful complex carbs and keep protein intake moderate.
- Snack healthfully throughout the day to stave off hunger pangs.
- Lower your fat intake to 20 percent or less of your daily calorie intake.

- Supplements—such as chromium picolinate, calcium, spirulina, and fat-burning appetite suppressants—can help you to lose and keep the weight off.
- Drink at least eight 8-ounce glasses of filtered or tap water daily, green tea, and low-cal, low-sodium beverages such as V-8 juice.
- Forget willpower—take control with a problem-solving approach.
- Exercise, exercise, exercise to boost your metabolism.
- Take advantage of low-fat, high carbs to feel calm and full.
- Watch your intake of refined carbos and raise your intake of quality low-fat protein to feel full and stave off hunger pangs.

Bios

Denise Bruner, M.D., is a bariatric physician and president of the American Society of Bariatric Physicians. She attended Howard University College of Medicine in Washington, D.C. She lives in Arlington, Virginia, is over 40, and has one child.

John P. Foreyt, Ph.D., went to Florida State University in Tallahassee graduate school and interned at University of Southern California medical school. He is a professor at Baylor College of Medicine in Houston, Texas; he sees patients and directs an obesity research clinic. He is the coauthor of *Living Without Dieting* (Warner Books), and at 58 he lives in Houston and is single.

Lisa Giannetto, M.D., is a doctor in associate medicine at the Duke University Medical Center, executive health program in Durham, North Carolina. She is also assistant clinical professor of medicine at Duke University. She received her medical degree at Loyola University Chicago–Stritch School of Medicine in Mainland, Illinois. She is 40, is married, and has two children.

Jan McBarron, M.D., a graduate of Hahnemann University in Philadelphia, Pennsylvania, is board certified in bariatric medicine. She is a specialist in preventive and weight loss medicine in Columbus, Georgia, where she has her practice and resides with her husband. She is the author of *Being a Woman Naturally: Dr. Jan McBarron's Guide to Natural Supplements Beyond 25* (Freedom Press). Web site: www.dukeandthedoctor.com.

Terry Shintani, M.D., M.P.H., received his M.P.H. in nutrition at Harvard University and his M.D. at the University of Hawaii. He is board certified in preventive medicine and is currently the director of preventive and integrative medicine at the Waianae Center in Honolulu, Hawaii. He practices integrative and nutritional medicine. He is author of *The Good Carbohydrate Revolution* (Pocket Books), *Dr. Shintani's Hawaii Diet* (Pocket Books), and *Dr. Shintani's Eat More, Weigh Less Diet* (Halpax). At 50, he is married, has two children, and lives in Honolulu.

Julian Whitaker, M.D., earned his medical degree at Emory University Medical School in Atlanta, Georgia. The director of the Whitaker Wellness Institute, he is the author of a variety of health books such as *Shed 10 Years in 10 Weeks* (Simon & Schuster) and Julian Whitaker—Health and Healing/Healthy Directions at www.phillips.com/health/catalog.htm. At 56, he is married, has eight children, and lives in Anaheim, California.

Judith Wurtman, Ph.D., received her Ph.D. from George Washington University in Washington, D.C. She is a research biochemist, is director of a weight management center at McLean Hospital in Boston, and has a clinic based on her research at MIT in Cambridge, Massachusetts. Dr. Wurtman is also coauthor of *The Serotonin Solution* (Fawcett Columbine). She is over 50, lives in Boston, is married, and has two children and three grandchildren. Web site: Triadwmc.org.

34

Pain

Q & A with Dr. Barnard

NEAL BARNARD, M.D.

The healing power of foods intrigues Neal Barnard, M.D., author of *Foods That Fight Pain* (Random House). He knows through his research that people suffer with arthritis, back pain, menstrual pain, and migraine headaches, never realizing that the cause could be what they eat—or don't eat.

When I spoke to Dr. Barnard he provided insight on food—something that I have been writing about for more than 15 years.

Q. *Did you have a personal experience with some type of pain and discover that food could provide relief?*
A. No. *Foods That Fight Pain* is for people with serious, chronic pain—for example, migraines that keep coming back or arthritis pain or back pain or fibromyalgia. I am delighted to say that, at least so far, I've been spared those kinds of problems.

Q. *You mention some principles in your book: pain-safe foods, soothing foods, and supplements if you need them. Explain.*
A. We want to identify foods that may be causing pain for us. For

migraine sufferers, for example, certain foods such as dairy products, chocolate, eggs, or citrus fruits can sometimes trigger the pain, as can certain beverages, red wine most commonly—and we want to avoid those. Second, sometimes there are foods that we can add to the diet to ease pain. Ginger can help some people; peppermint oil can help with stomach pain. So we add them if we need to.

Q. *According to your book, you break it up into different pain problems. Can you give me an example of how this works?*
A. With regard to circulatory conditions, we think of heart disease, and the chest pain that can come from it, as very different from back pain. The fact is, they may very well have a common denominator. If you block off the blood supply to the heart you risk a heart attack. If you block off the blood supply to the lower back you choke off the blood supply to the discs, which are the cushions between the vertebrae. When they lose their blood supply they become fragile and they can then burst. And that's what is behind much of the lower back pain, which is such an epidemic.

So the answer in both cases is to follow a diet and lifestyle that open those arteries up again. Dr. Dean Ornish did some wonderful pioneering research on opening up the arteries to the heart. And the good news is, if you do that it's quite likely you'll keep the arteries open in the rest of the body as well.

Q. *What about food sensitivities?*
A. Migraines are a perfect example of food sensitivities. This doesn't mean you're allergic in the same way a person might have a rash from eating strawberries. But it does mean that the food triggers the pain. When a person identifies their trigger and avoids that food, they will often feel better.

Q. *How about hormonal-related pain like monthly killer menstrual cramps?*
A. A change in diet can be absolutely a lifesaver. When you cut the fat in your diet, the hormones shift. As you're smoothing out those hormonal shifts, menstrual pain can drop just as cravings can be diminished as well.

The most helpful diet for doing these things is a low-fat vegan diet, meaning a pure vegetarian diet because it doesn't have any animal products in it at all so there's no animal fat. [Dr. Barnard is a strict vegetarian.] If we keep the vegetable oils low, too, then we really knock out the fat that causes these hormone aberrations to occur.

Q. *What about metabolic and immune problems—how can food help?*
A. If we look at different conditions such as diabetes or carpal tunnel syndrome we find that by choosing our foods more selectively we can sometimes knock out these problems. With diabetes, again it's a low-fat vegan diet that you want, with fiber-rich foods that cause the insulin in the body to work a little better. For carpal tunnel syndrome, this repetitive motion condition, some people have gotten benefits from vitamin B_6. The dose that is typically used in these research studies is about 50 to 150 milligrams per day. So there is a variety of diet; that was the message of *Foods That Fight Pain.*

Q. *What about herpes and shingles?*
A. We carry viruses that can either remain dormant or kick in with a cold sore. When the cold sore goes away it doesn't mean the virus is gone—it just means that it's gone into remission. It means that your immune system has tackled it. It's good if we have certain foods in our diet that keep a strong immune system functioning. If you avoid fatty foods and animal products especially, because cholesterol can harm the immune system, you're going to be better off. If you have a diet rich in vegetables and fruits, you'll get beta carotene and vitamin C—those are immune boosters. A lot of us don't get enough of those in our diet and you want to bring them back.

Q. *Why do activity, rest, and diet help make our aches and pains seem less painful?*
A. If we're tired, everything hurts worse. Psychological hurts affect us more—we're more irritable; and physical hurts bother us, too. If we get on a healthy cycle, exercise during the day, sleep at

night, then everything seems to go better. If a person has pain, you want to change your diet.

Q. *What is the most healthful diet plan?*
A. In my opinion, that's a low-fat vegan diet, rich in vegetables and fruits. Take a multivitamin to cover yourself for any vitamins you might be low in. Add daily exercise. Start with a half-hour walk every day. See your doctor if you have any kind of health condition. But gradually increase and really enjoy how it feels to be in a good, healthy, vigorous body.

Q. *We're talking about food to cure pain, but isn't it easier to take painkillers?*
A. Easier yes, but more effective no. If I take a painkiller maybe it will knock out my headache for a while, but it will come back. Maybe you can knock out menstrual pain, but you're going to have it again the next month. If you change your diet to prevent these things it's better than all the painkillers in the world.

THE DOC'S SUPPLEMENT LIST

Here are some of the supplements that Dr. Barnard believes can help fight pain.

Supplement	What It Does
Beta carotene	Beta carotene, which is converted into vitamin A, has antioxidant effects that can boost the immune system
Vitamin B$_6$	This vitamin can help prevent the pain of carpal tunnel syndrome
Vitamin C	An immune-boosting antioxidant vitamin that can help fight autoimmune health problems such as shingles and herpes

Ginger	An herbal remedy that can help fight nausea and vomiting
Peppermint oil	Oil capsules can help soothe stomach problems (such as gas and nausea)

Safety Smarts: Vitamin C: If you take too much, it can cause gastrointestinal problems. Peppermint: Too much can cause heartburn.

DOC'S RX TO HEAL YOURSELF

- Avoid trigger foods that can cause pain.
- Follow a heart-healthy diet and lifestyle.
- Eat a low-fat, vegetarian-based diet to prevent hormonal-related pain.
- Opt for vitamin B supplements to prevent and treat carpal tunnel syndrome pain.
- Eat fewer fatty foods and animal products and more immune-boosting fruits and vegetables, which are chock-full of antioxidant nutrients.

BIO

Neal Barnard, M.D., is president of the Committee of Physicians for Responsible Medicine in Washington, D.C. He attended George Washington University. At 47, his specialty is psychiatry; he sees patients solely in research studies. He lives in Washington, D.C. Web site: www.drbarnard.com.

35

Aging

FOUNTAIN OF YOUTH WITH DR. FOX

ARNOLD FOX, M.D.

From the first moment I spoke with Dr. Arnold Fox, I could tell he is a practicing preventive doctor from the old school. By that I mean that this senior doc cares about the well-being of his patients. And as a senior physician he exudes enthusiasm with a capital *E*.

When Dr. Fox sees new patients, he uses his craft like a sly fox to find out their philosophy about health—"because if it doesn't include taking care of themselves, we're wasting our time unless I can convert them into thinking about health as the main role," he explains.

His main interest, these days, is setting up a lifetime preventive health program for his patients of all ages. He troubleshoots different problems. For instance, "They're young and say, 'I feel wonderful and I don't want to be like my mother or father who is always ill. What can you do?' or they'll say, 'I feel tired all the time. And the other doctors say, "You're getting older—you're 50 or 60." Is that true?' I say, 'No it's not true. You should feel good,' because I want them to feel as good as I do. And at 73 I feel very, very good," says Dr. Fox. So he puts his patients on a five-part program, which he, a healthy senior, follows himself.

1. Eat a berry healthful diet. Dr. Fox eats a low-fat, nutrient-dense diet. His usual breakfast is a fruit shake with a variety of fresh berries and other fruit, nonfat milk, and ice cubes. "Blueberries especially have a profound effect upon vision," he points out. His radio talk show listeners vow that their eye doctors have seen a difference after they eat blueberries regularly for six months. "For lunch I usually have a big salad and a couple of vegetables. For dinner, three or four nights a week it's a big piece of salmon and three to four vegetables. I must have four to five vegetables a day and at least three pieces of fruit."

2. Exercise! Dr. Fox works out every day, which is an inspiration to both young and old. "I like going to the club because I have a regular routine. On the treadmill it's 40 minutes (I start it at 3.7 mph and I work up to 4.4 mph usually at a 1 percent grade); and I go through nine or ten machines—not heavy weights," he told me. "I look around me, and my friends who graduated from high school when I did, in 1946, are on canes and insulin."

3. Stay positive. "Maintain total enthusiasm," he says. "I don't know if you can tell by my voice how enthusiastic I am to be talking to you, but I talk to everyone this way—especially patients. I made a bet with a patient and said, 'If you ever catch me in a down mood, ask me for ten dollars and I'll give it to you.' Enthusiasm will get you over the bumps in the road of life and it has a beneficial effect upon your life. Enthusiastic people are much healthier than depressed, cynical, and angry people."

4. Supplement your diet. A past mentor-doctor influenced Dr. Fox because his patients were always healthier than everybody else and never had a complication. He was doing things like writing on the patients' medical charts "no canned food, no processed food, no sugar." The dietitians hated him, recalls Dr. Fox. "The doctors hated him because

he wrote on the charts (this was the 1960s) 'zinc, vitamin C, B complex.' I took careful records for one year of all the patients that I was seeing from other doctors and I came to the conclusion that whatever he was doing was working for his patients." And Dr. Fox soon began to follow in his supplement-savvy mentor's footsteps.

5. Take hormones. For men and women patients Dr. Fox checks a whole gamut of hormones from testosterone to progesterone. Then he will discuss with his patient, "Should you take hormones? If you have any reason not to, then you shouldn't. If there is a cancer of the prostate or a cancer of the reproductive system in women, then you probably shouldn't take it." However, as an alternative healing doc, he does believe in natural hormones for well-being and takes hormonal supplements himself.

After discussing Dr. Fox's anti-aging strategies, I couldn't help asking "Are you healthy?" He replied, "Am I healthy? My grandchildren say, 'The other grandfathers are old and yet they're younger than you. They can't run like you.' I'm not superman, but I have tremendous energy. What I want for my patients is what I have for myself. I want them to be energetic and have a productive life."

AGING MYTHS

Myths such as those quoted below only waste a striving senior's time, money, and energy. Here's to wisdom (and young-at-heart Dr. Fox, who inspired me) and dispelling the aging mystique.

Myth 1. If young is beautiful, old must be unattractive.
Fact. Remember, inner beauty cuts beneath the surface (of gray hair, wrinkles, or flab) and real candor shines through. Personal traits (character, intelligence, and social skills) are attractive at any age. Open your eyes—we have a lot of role models in this book who are over 50 and look great.

Myth 2. Seniors are sexless.

Fact. Many people still think that libido plummets after 50. (Check out the next chapter if you are feeling desexed.) But, experts say, that's simply untrue. According to a Kinsey Institute Report on Sex, 70 percent of married men over 65 have sexual relations, and men and women who were sexually active in youth are likely to be sexually active seniors.

Myth 3. Older people are useless in the workplace.

Fact. Although downsizing is a reality, it happens because older employees tend to be more costly than younger workers. Yet research indicates eliminating older workers may backfire. Also, if you take a look at the median age of the 101 doctors in this book it's mid-fifties.

Myth 4. Elders are senile, ill, and useless.

Fact. "Despite our fears that the aging brain must fall prey to senility, the vast majority of old people retain their faculties intact and many creative abilities ripen toward the very end of life," says *Ageless Body Timeless Mind* (Harmony Books) author Deepak Chopra, M.D.

THE DOC'S SUPPLEMENT LIST

Here are just *some* of the favorite anti-aging supplements that Dr. Fox takes himself, and also recommends to his patients (however, the dosage differs for each individual).

Supplement	What It Does	Dose
Alpha-lipoic acid	A fantastic antioxidant that goes into the cell and around the cell; recharges antioxidants vitamin C and E	333 mg per day
B complex 100	Lowers homocysteine, which can reduce stroke and Alzheimer's disease	100 mg twice a day

Vitamin C	Super anti–heart disease antioxidant; it's an immune system stimulant and kills viruses; boosts energy	5,000 mg twice a day
DHEA	It is an anti-aging hormone.	50 mg per day
Vitamin E	Superb antioxidant that decreases free radical damage.	400 IU twice a day
L-carnitine	An amino acid that affects the triglycerides, keeping the "bad" cholesterol down; takes fat into cells where it can be burnt for energy	500 mg per day

Safety Smarts: Alpha-lipoic acid: If you are diabetic and taking insulin, lipoic acid can lower your blood glucose level, which may lower your need for medications. Talk to your doctor. Vitamin C: If you take too much, it can cause gastrointestinal problems.

DR. WERBACH'S LONGEVITY POINTERS

MELVYN WERBACH, M.D.

When I asked Dr. Melvyn Werbach, "What is the one longevity strategy that you wouldn't want to do without?" he answered, "Personal satisfaction." I pressed: "No, something to help keep you healthy." And he repeated, "Something that would be personally satisfying." So I listened.

"It could be building or studying. It could be relating to somebody intimately. There is a lot of scientific evidence that personal satisfaction links to longevity," he says. And personal satisfaction can rev up those feel-good endorphins, lower blood pressure, and boost the immune system.

Meanwhile, like the other doctors in this book, Dr. Werbach exercises regularly and eats right to stall Father Time.

THE DOC'S SUPPLEMENT LIST

Dr. Werbach also takes these anti-aging supplements to boost his good health and longevity.

Supplement	What It Does
Ginkgo biloba	An herb that aids in preventing loss of memory
Vitamin C	An antioxidant that strengthens the immune system
Multivitamin-and-mineral supplement	Ensures getting adequate vitamins and minerals for optimal health
Omega-3 fatty acids	Essential fatty acids help to provide adequate amount of good fats in the diet
Soy powder	Protein supplement that contains isoflavones, which inhibit cancers; aids in prostate health

Safety Smarts: Ginkgo biloba: Do not take more than 240 milligrams; it may cause dermatitis, diarrhea, and vomiting. Do not use it with blood-thinning medications, aspirin, or NSAIDs (nonsteroidal anti-inflammatory medicines). Vitamin C: If you take too much, it can cause gastrointestinal problems. Omega-3 oils: Don't take high doses of fish oil capsules if you are taking NSAIDs. It may increase gastrointestinal ulcers and bleeding.

LONGEVITY TIPS FROM
DRS. BLUMBERG, BENEDIKT, AND HUNGERLAND

JEFFREY BLUMBERG, PH.D.

I have interviewed Dr. Jeffrey Blumberg for many years on the topic on antioxidant vitamins. It seemed natural to ask the doctor, "What is *your* favorite vitamin?"

Without hesitation he told me: "It's simple—vitamin E. It's because getting the optimal intake of vitamin E is probably impossible through diet, so you need some supplemental help," he told me.

Evidence suggests that vitamin E helps to promote good health. For example, it benefits immune responses and reduces the risk of chronic diseases like cataracts, heart disease, and some forms of cancer. It's an easy answer because we have more data about vitamin E than most any other antioxidants, explains Dr. Blumberg.

However, he adds, "Vitamin E is a problematic nutrient. Clearly it is an important and essential antioxidant. But it is really found only in high-fat foods—vegetable oils like margarine, salad dressing, nuts (almonds), and wheat germ. It is associated with a good amount of calories if you eat a lot of it. I'm not suggesting that you can't incorporate those foods as part of a healthful diet— and you should do so." But the fact remains, Dr. Blumberg does not want to live on large quantities of salad dressing.

"The reason that vitamin E is my favorite, and not vitamin C, is because I eat a lot of citrus fruits, and I drink a lot of orange juice. And so it's not as important as a supplement because I get it in my diet," says Dr. Blumberg.

HOWARD BENEDIKT, D.C.

Dr. Howard Benedikt, like many of his colleagues, is very enthusiastic about looking at what can be done not only to intervene and help in well-being, but to find things people can do to reverse the aging process.

So what does Dr. Benedikt do to live longer and healthier?

- *Gets adequate sleep.* "It's so important. It gives your body an opportunity to deal with repairing the breakdown of your cells (due to stress, hormones, exposure to the environment, and so on) on a daily basis," he says.
- *Manages his stress.* "I learned to put everything into perspective. Every day I take five minutes from my schedule to relax and close my eyes and get into a state of total relaxation," he says. "It's very relaxing to go for a walk and have my mind off of things. For me it's walking and treadmill three times a week. Studies have shown that exercise reduces stress. It helps burn calories. It is a physical activity to help you maintain an ideal weight."
- *Avoids alcohol and nicotine.* While Dr. Benedikt doesn't drink alcohol or smoke, he points out that there are studies that have shown that drinking red wine is beneficial because of the antioxidants in it. "But I would turn around and say you can get these antioxidants in your diet and in supplemental form," he says.
- *Watches his diet.* He eats a low-carbohydrate, moderate-protein, and desirable-fat diet: 40 percent complex carbs, 30 percent desirable fat, and 30 percent protein. "The goal is to keep you in the zone so you don't have elevations of insulin. Eating too many carbohydrates—as the American public is prone to do because they don't want to eat a lot of animal protein—converts those carbohydrates into fat. And that's why obesity is such a big issue here in the United States. You need to have more complex carbohydrate."

THE DOC'S SUPPLEMENT LIST

Dr. Benedikt uses these supplements in his stay-young health plan.

Supplement	What It Does
Multivitamin-and-mineral supplement	Aids in getting adequate vitamins and minerals in your daily diet to enhance optimal health
Antioxidant formula	Enhances the total body to prevent age-related diseases
Vitamin C	Boosts the immune system to stave off heart disease and cancer
Omega-3 fatty acids	Essential fatty acids enhance the overall diet, especially if you don't eat enough fish

Safety Smarts: Vitamin C can cause gastrointestinal problems if you take too much. Omega-3 oils: Don't take high doses of fish oil if you are taking NSAIDs (nonsteroidal anti-inflammatory drugs). It may increase gastrointestinal ulcers and bleeding.

JACKLYN HUNGERLAND, PH.D.

Retired psychologist Jacklyn Hungerland, Ph.D., a senior, stays active, limber, and upbeat. What helps to keep her young, she told me, helps her to feel good. The anti-aging prescription? Her dogs!

We know our dog companions are affectionate and their presence is comforting, but according to Dr. Hungerland, dogs can do much more than comfort us. She feels that spending time with dogs is largely what has kept her young in mind, spirit, and body.

Although she's retired from the board of the American Kennel

Club, Hungerland still judges at dog shows. "The traveling is the difficult part," she says, "but it's so reinforcing. Each show is an exciting adventure. It's like being on stage. It boosts the ego." An added bonus is that she "gets to play with everybody else's dogs," with no strings attached.

She currently lives with two black poodles (a standard and a miniature) and a Bouvier des Flandres. Her comforting canines provide psychological and physical benefits that contribute to her feelings of well-being. Seven years ago, for instance, Dr. Hungerland underwent open-chest surgery to remedy pleurisy (in which the double membrane, or pleura, that lines the chest cavity and surrounds the lungs becomes inflamed). While recovering in the hospital she felt a lump in her breast—and that's how the doctors discovered that she had breast cancer. "I was pretty overwhelmed," she admitted, but survived the double whammy—thanks to canine support.

One day while she was recuperating at home, the doctor's dogs paid her an unforgettable visit. They went into the upstairs room "tiptoeing," she recalls, "and sat quietly. They treated me the same way they treat people in the convalescent hospital."

Dr. Hungerland, a dog person since she was four, believes that most people, whether raised in the city or the country, can relate to dogs. "It takes them back to that youthful spring," she says, "that inner spiritual spring of happiness and comfort."

DOCS' RX TO HEAL YOURSELF

- Eat a nutrient-rich diet to keep your optimal health.
- Exercise to maintain a healthy and energetic body.
- Stay positive to live a healthier and longer life.
- Supplement your diet with anti-aging supplements such as alpha-lipoic acid, vitamin B complex, vitamin A, L-carnitine, ginkgo biloba, omega-3 fatty acids, soy powder, and more.
- Get adequate sleep, destress, and avoid alcohol and nicotine.
- Use pet therapy for its healing powers.

BIOS

Howard Benedikt, D.C., received his doctorate of chiropractic from the National College of Chiropractic in Lombard, Illinois. He is board certified in anti-aging therapeutics and is on the board of directors of the American Academy of Antiaging Health Practitioners in Chicago, Illinois. At 51, he has been in clinical practice for 25 years and works in New York City. Web site: DrBenedikt.com.

Jeffrey Blumberg, Ph.D., is professor of nutrition at Tufts University in Boston, Massachusetts. He graduated from Vanderbilt Medical School. He lives in Newton, Massachusetts. He is 56, is married, and has two sons.

Arnold Fox, M.D., is a 73-year-old practicing physician, internist/cardiologist, and anti-aging specialist in Los Angeles, California. He received his M.D. from the University of California at Irvine and was on the faculty of UCI for about 20 years. He is the coauthor of several health-related books such as *The Fat Blocker Diet* (St. Martin's Press) and coauthor (along with Barry Fox, Ph.D.) of *Alternative Healing* (Career Press). Dr. Fox resides in Woodland Hills, has been married for 50 years, and has seven children.

Jacklyn Hungerland, Ph.D., graduated from the United States International University in San Diego. She is a retired psychologist whose past part-time practice included visits to a skilled nursing facility with one of her pooches. At 70, she has a son and daughter, four grandchildren, and three great grandchildren.

Melvyn Werbach, M.D., is a full-time doctor who specializes in nutrition. He received his M.D. from Tufts University in Boston, Massachusetts. He is the author of *The Nutritional Influences on Illness* (Third Line Press). At 60, he is married, has two children, and lives and works in Tarzana, California.

36

Sexual Health

DR. WATSON'S LOVE POTIONS

CYNTHIA WATSON, M.D.

Sex is a good preventive health medicine. Sex provides many health benefits, from reducing pain to stimulating the body's circulation. So how can you jump-start your libido? Just ask Cynthia Watson, M.D., author of *Love Potions* (Tarcher/Putnam), how to "trick" your body into feeling sexier. She shares her healthy strategies on how to preserve a healthy sex drive.

- *Eat a low-fat, nutrient-dense diet.* Dr. Watson fills her plate with healthy, low-fat foods, which is the prescription for sexual vitality, potency, and health. Not only will it help keep off body fat, it will make you feel healthy and sexy. "Today I had cottage cheese and bananas for breakfast, and green-bean-and-asparagus salad with sesame dressing and a piece of fish at lunch. For dinner I'll probably have a salad," she told me.

  "You don't want to eat foods that are heavy in fat and hard to digest. You want to keep your arteries clean and really nourish your body. My philosophy is that I should be an example for my patients. I believe in staying well and healthy and keeping myself vital as I age. How can I teach other people to do the things that I think they should do to stay healthy if I'm not showing them that it can be done?"

- *Do cardiovascular exercise.* She dances (jazz) an hour and a half three times a week. "It keeps me in such good shape and it's such a creative outlet. It makes me feel sexy. It makes me feel very beautiful to dance," says Dr. Watson. Cardiovascular exercise (jogging, swimming, or aerobics such as dancing) alters metabolic rate, often resulting in a greater sense of well-being, energy, and confidence—all natural aphrodisiacs.

Dr. Watson, who sees both female and male patients regularly, knows that eating more nutrient-rich foods—containing vitamins A, B complex, and E and zinc—can enhance sexual health.

"They boost good health, which helps provide better sexual energy," says Dr. Watson. "The sex drive requires a balance between the endocrine and neurologic systems, and the foods that are the most sexually stimulating contain nutrients that support these systems."

Holistically speaking, sexual intimacy can help maintain a healthy mind, body, and spirit. Good sex can not only make people feel better physically, but also uplift their spirits and boost positive thinking.

"Sex with love can reassure and relieve men and women of their deepest fears and anxieties, free them to be themselves, and if Eastern thinkers are right, lead them to a higher plane of consciousness," says Dr. Watson. "There are also Western sages who basically agree that loving sexuality is a pathway to the meaning of life."

LIBIDO AND LIFESTYLE

Medical experts like Dr. Watson recommend following these passion pointers to enhance your sexual desire:

- *Stay away from dairy products.* This is especially important if you're trying to boost your sexual energy. Milk before bed ensures a good night's sleep, not an orgasm.
- *Slice the fat from your diet.* Researchers have found that fatty meals curb the production of testosterone, a hormone that affects sex drive. Plus, fat clogs arteries—including those leading to the penis.
- *Cut back on alcohol.* It can depress the desire and ability to perform.
- *Review your medications.* Certain medications interfere with sex drive and greatly influence potency. Check with your doctor if you're taking diet pills, antihistamines, ulcer medications, decongestants, or antidepressants.
- *Chill out.* Just lowering blood pressure can positively affect the desire to make love. Regular exercise, meditation, and vacations may be the best aphrodisiacs of all.

THE DOC'S SUPPLEMENT LIST

Here are some of the love nutrients that Dr. Watson takes herself and recommends to patients, which can bring out a man and woman's sensual side.

Supplement	How It Works
Vitamin A	Antioxidant, contains precursor to testosterone
Vitamin B complex	Calms nerves. The nervous system is stimulated when you're sexually aroused; you need well-functioning nerves
Vitamin C	Antioxidant that may boost circulation to genital area; keeps your skin, hair, and nails healthy
Vitamin E	Antioxidant believed to be a sex vitamin; makes hormones

Multivitamin-and-mineral supplement	To get adequate vitamins and minerals in a busy life
Zinc	Mineral inhibits damage to the body system that produces dopamine, a neurotransmitter linked with feelings of well-being and libido

Safety Smarts: Vitamin A: It can be toxic in large amounts (more than 10,000 IU) since it's stored in the liver. Vitamin C: If you take too much, it can cause gastrointestinal problems.

RESEARCH IN A NUTSHELL

A study of men suffering from mild to moderate lagging libido known as "erectile dysfunction" found their sexual performance was enhanced after taking ginkgo biloba, American and Korean ginseng, the amino acid L-arginine, and vitamins A, C, E, and B complex and the minerals selenium and zinc.

The research showed that a month of supplements improved the ability to maintain an erection in 90 percent of ten men. Nearly half were more satisfied with their sex life. (Ito TY, Kawahara K, Das AK, Strudwick W. "A pilot study on the effects of ArginMax, a natural dietary supplement for enhancement of male sexual function." *Hawaii Medical Journal*, 1998; 57 (12:741– 774).

DEFYING AGE WITH DR. LAMM

STEVEN LAMM, M.D.

"If the mission is to have great sex, you need to balance your physical and emotional state. In order to experience great sex, you have to be in tiptop physiologic condition," Dr. Steven Lamm told me.

Simply put, good heart function, good muscle function, good flexibility, and blood vessels that are clear of plaque will enhance blood flow to the genital organs, says internist Stephen Lamm, M.D., the author of *The Virility Solution* (Simon & Schuster).

So how does Dr. Lamm keep his libido healthy? The most important things Dr. Lamm does to keep sexually healthy are as follows:

- *Have a caring partner.* "You have to have a partner that you're committed to and that you can share feelings with," says Dr. Lamm. Keep in mind, men and women have different needs (it's possible males are more physiologically driven and women may have not only a physiologic requirement but also an intimacy requirement, points out Dr. Lamm). That means if you want to have great sex you have to understand the basic needs of your partner—and meet their needs, adds Dr. Lamm.
- *Feel a sense of well-being.* "You have to feel good about yourself; then you feel entitled to have great sex," he says. This, in turn, means you have to take care of your body.
- *Exercise regularly.* Dr. Lamm turns to weight training and jumping rope. It's a one-hour program at least four times a week. Some days it's a combination of both activities. "It helps cardiovascular status and muscles, which stimulates not only endorphins but probably testosterone production," he says.
- *Eat a nutrient-dense diet.* Dr. Lamm's diet is rich in antioxidants because he eats plenty of fruits and vegetables. "It's the only way you can preserve the integrity of your blood vessels and enhance blood flow," he explains. That's important for both men and women in enhancing orgasms.

THE DOC'S SUPPLEMENT LIST

Here are the libido-boosting supplements that Dr. Lamm recommends:

Supplement	What It Does
Multivitamin-and-mineral supplement	For general good health and well-being.
Pycnogenol	This antioxidant protects the blood vessels, which can help sustain erections.
Selenium	This antioxidant trace mineral is for good prostate health. An enlarged prostate puts pressure on your bladder, so you don't want to have a chronic disorder, because it will dampen your libido.
Soy	It's a protein supplement that contains isoflavones, which inhibit cancers; good for a healthy prostate.

Safety Smarts: Selenium: Too much (more than 600 mcg per day) can be harmful.

STAYING HEALTHY WITH SEX

Surprise! Doctors claim that an active love life is a prescription for good health. Here are five reasons to postpone sexual retirement:

1. Sex bolsters the immune system. Studies show that any pleasurable activity can increase the number and effectiveness of infection-fighting cells in the immune system, ac-

cording to coauthors Dr. David Weeks and Jamie James in their book *Secrets of the Superyoung* (Villard).

2. Sex staves off insomnia. According to a National Sleep Foundation poll, 56 percent of mature adults report one symptom of insomnia. The good news is that many people have discovered an effective, natural way to get rid of tension before bedtime. A little romance may prove more effective than a cup of milk. The big payoff? During sexual activity, the brain produces endorphins, which have a soothing, relaxing effect on the body—especially after orgasm.

3. Sex reduces pain. These same endorphins—nature's pain relievers—are able to circulate throughout the body and ease various types of pain. Sexual activity, therefore, may offer relief to arthritis sufferers. Again, the answer may be in the effects of yes, yes—orgasm.

4. Sex subtracts years. "Improving the quality of one's sex life can help a person to look between four and seven years younger," claim coauthors Dr. Weeks and James. The reason? Less stress, more contentment.

5. Sex boosts longevity. The consensus is that a healthy, active sex life stalls and prevents age-related physical and psychological problems. What's more, studies at the Institute for Advanced Study of Human Sexuality in San Francisco show that a gratifying love life enhances success and happiness outside the bedroom, too.

RELATIONSHIP TIPS FROM DRS. MCCARTHY AND GREER

BARRY MCCARTHY, PH.D.

Here is Dr. Barry McCarthy's personal message to us on how he keeps his marriage happy and healthy:

Sex and intimacy keep me healthy for two reasons. One of the rituals my wife and I have is a 45-minute walk each morning. It's our favorite way to stay connected. Sometimes we do it for fun and sometimes to catch up on things. I work in Washington Monday through Thursday, so it's our way of reconnecting. It keeps the head clear, it's a physically healthy thing to do, and it's a psychological way to stay connected.

I'm a big fan theoretically, clinically, and personally of having a regular rhythm of being connected. One of the things I always write about, and try to practice in my own life, is to try not to go two weeks (at the absolute maximum) without some sort of a sexual connection. Our ritual is to take this walk and then go and have breakfast, then go home, take a shower, and be sexual. The notion about sexuality is that you want to set up a rhythm where you stay connected in your relationship. It's an energizer both in terms of you as a person and your bond. It's one of the things that keeps you as a person and your relationship vital and healthy.

JANE GREER, PH.D.

Communication is vital to a healthy relationship. Dr. Jane Greer, who has been married for 19 years, knows firsthand that this fact is true. "Communication is the bridge that helps partners connect with each other in order to feel understood and accepted," she says.

"The key to good communication is to talk about the way you wind up feeling in the time somebody says or does something that they may or may not have intended to do," explains Dr. Greer. This, in turn, gives them an opportunity to relate to the fact that they made you feel bad and shed light on what their actual intention was.

Dr. Greer offers these six good communication tips:

1. Listen, without giving solutions or problem-solving, to what the other person is sharing.
2. When your mate is talking about how hard their day is or

how much they have to do, empathize without talking about your own pressures.

3. Be supportive and nonjudgmental with what they share with you.
4. Avoid criticism and blame.
5. Preserve respect by talking respectfully.
6. Be playful and use your sense of humor.

Doc's Rx to Heal Yourself

- Eat a low-fat, nutrient-dense diet for good health and sexual vitality.
- Exercise to feel healthy, confident, and sexy.
- Avoid culprits—dairy, fat, alcohol, certain medications, and stress—that can dampen your sex drive.
- Opt for libido-boosting antioxidants—such as vitamins A, C, and E, and selenium—and take B complex for optimal sexual health.
- Take pycnogenol and soy to maintain a healthy prostate.
- Stay connected with your partner and practice good communication.

Bios

Jane Greer, P.h.D., is a marriage and sex therapist who practices in New York City. She received her Ph.D. at Adelphi University, Garden City, New York. She is the author of *How Could You Do This to Me?* and *Gridlock: Finding the Courage to Move On in Love, Work and Life* (both by Doubleday). She is over 40 and married. Web site: www.DrJaneGreer.com.

Steven Lamm, M.D., is an internist who went to New York University Medical Center. He is the author of *The Virility Solution* (Simon & Schuster). He has a private practice in New York City. At 52, he is married and has five children.

Barry McCarthy, Ph.D., is a psychologist (sex therapy is his subspecialty) at Washington Psychological Center in Washington, D.C. He has a Ph.D. in psychology from Southern Illinois University. He is the coauthor of *Couples Sexual Awareness* and *Male Sexual Awareness* (both Carroll & Graf). At 57, he is married, lives in Wilmington, Delaware, and has three children and one grandchild.

Cynthia Watson, M.D., is board certified in family practice and is a clinical instructor in the department of family medicine at the University of Southern California school of medicine, where she received her M.D. At 50, she is a mother and practices with an emphasis on herbal, homeopathic, and nutritional medicine in Santa Monica, California. Web site: Cynthiawatson.com.

37

Environmental Toxins

Dr. Haas's Detox Diet

ELSON M. HAAS, M.D.

Dr. Elson Haas takes pride in being tagged as "the lifestyle doctor." And he personally practices what he preaches: preventive medicine. That includes nutrition, exercise, sleep, stress management. And those components are the basis of the choices we make in the way we live.

"My therapeutic approach is lifestyle first, natural medicine second, and drugs last," he told me and discussed it in detail from his home office.

On The Detox Diet *book*

"It's very simple, it's a basic concept. It gives a how-to program on getting people off SNACC—which stands for sugar, nicotine, alcohol, caffeine, and chemicals. Almost every American is hooked into one of those substances."

On Detoxification—the missing link in the American diet

"When I graduated from medical school I was 50 pounds overweight and I had allergies every day. I was introduced to a man who taught me about cleansing and I went on a juice cleanse for ten days. On the third day my head was clear and my allergies were gone. And all I was doing was drinking lemonade. Over that ten days my body got rid of water weight, I shifted almost 20 pounds. I realized what I was putting in my body was much more than I needed. It's about choices. In that time, it was 1975, I changed my diet. I realized I was going to choose healthy, vibrant foods from the earth primarily as my nutrition. I lost 45 pounds over that year."

On the detoxification process

"During the middle of it I felt so incredibly well and clear. I was sleeping less. My body felt the way I wanted it to feel forever. I just felt so good. I got rid of half of my stuff—all the junk that was sitting around me. I started my life fresh and new. And that's when I realized I wanted to change how health care is delivered. I want to teach people how to take care of themselves."

On how his detoxification process works

"It just helps your body's system catch up to the present. Our body is used to creating waste and getting rid of it. If we don't have any waste going into our mouths over a period of time, our bodies will get rid of the waste that's in the tissues in different parts of the body and our body will start to feel lighter. It's the waste products, the toxicity, the congestion in the body that leads to a lot of aches and pains, inflammation, and aging that people experience. I have seen all kinds of medical problems and symptoms in myself and in thousands of patients over the years that get better when they stop taking toxins and flush their systems: drinking more water, eating more fresh fruits and vegetables, juices and certain herbs that stimulate the liver to detoxify, and various things."

On his patients who detox their lifestyles

"Lately I have been doing detox groups. I'm getting a lot more people that are coming in for that. And my books tell people how to do it. I have people look into their habits: 'Okay, what I am hooked into? What am I overdoing?' Would you consider taking a break? That's the message of *The Detox Diet*. Taking a break from anything that you're doing on a daily basis that you feel dependent on for energy or relaxation. That's caffeine and alcohol very commonly."

On the most common pollutants people are addicted to

"Just chemical foods and processed wheats and fats—the things that clog up the system. These are what I call the congesting kinds of foods."

On natural medicine

"Natural medicine works to rebuild the body. We use natural things. We use the right molecules and the right dosages. The idea of functional medicine is that we evaluate the function of the body and we get it working optimally. We give it all the right nutrients—fatty acids, amino acids, minerals and vitamins to support the health. And that's what I do personally as well. I watch my body—how it feels. And if I feel like I'm getting sluggish or clogged up or my allergies start to come up a little bit—this is over 25 years that I have had minimal allergies—if I sweep the garage or mow the lawn I'll sneeze. But I used to be allergic all the time."

On detoxification withdrawal symptoms

"If you do it properly with water and nutrients and the Detox Diet, which is an alkalizing diet, you don't get as many symptoms. But if you drink coffee every day you're almost sure to get a headache. Sugar—no. Alcohol—it can be."

On his current diet behavior

"I do a ten-day juice cleanse every spring—just like the first time 26 years ago. But now I have learned. I have 20, 30, or 40 patients do it along with me. It motivates me to do it because everyone is going to try it."

On a sample of the juice cleanse diet

"You could do a cleanse, which is the same thing every day. You just drink Master Cleanser, which is a lemonade formula: 2 tablespoons of fresh lemon juice, 1 tablespoon of maple syrup, $\frac{1}{10}$ tablespoon of cayenne pepper (good-quality red pepper), and 8 ounces of water. Drink eight to ten glasses a day. And there are other factors such as getting your bowels working; drinking other water, herb teas; what substances are okay and not okay."

On including dietary supplements with the detoxification diet

"I didn't used to but now I do occasionally such as blue-green algae or chlorella with amino acids for my brain."

On motivation

"Attitude is the underlying basis of all preventive medicine because you've got to be motivated to take care of yourself in a positive, loving way. And that's what I learned for myself. Before, I used to be more self-destructive and unconscious. Now I have learned what makes me feel better. That's what I do on a daily basis and what I encourage my patients to do. Pay attention to what you are doing and how you feel, and when you change it, if you feel better that's a message to you that it's probably better for your body."

Dr. Rountree's Superfoods for Kids

ROBERT ROUNTREE, M.D.

One of the biggest problems children face is the invisible but steadily increasing danger of exposure to heavy metals and organic toxins found in contaminated food and water, according to Robert Rountree, M.D., author of *Smart Medicine for a Healthier Child* and *Parent's Guide to Medical Emergencies* (both published by Avery Publishing Group).

"These toxins are being referred to by experts as POPs (persistent organic pollutants). More and more research shows that long-term exposure to such toxins (which in this generation starts in the womb) puts children at risk for developing a wide range of illnesses including cancer, autoimmune disease, allergy, asthma, and recurrent infections from weak immune systems," says Dr. Rountree.

He adds, "The best overall way that I know of to boost children's health is to have them eat organically grown foods and to include lots of detoxifying 'superfoods' in their diet, which helps to bolster their resistance against the onslaught of toxins." Here, Dr. Rountree lists nine types of foods that help guard your children against illness:

1. Berries (blueberries, strawberries, raspberries). Rich in antioxidant flavonoid pigments such as anthocyanidins, resveratrol, and ellagic acid. Support the immune system by neutralizing free radicals (molecules that destroy normal cells and cause degenerative diseases such as cancer).
2. Citrus fruits (oranges, grapefruit). High in vitamin C and bioflavonoids, which are immune-boosting.
3. Turmeric and rosemary. Contain disease-fighting antioxidants.
4. Green tea. Another antioxidant-rich source that makes an excellent alternative to synthetic, sugar-based chemical drinks like Coke and Kool-Aid.
5. Colorful vegetables (bell peppers, tomatoes, winter squashes,

sweet potatoes). Rich in carotene compounds, which are another family of food-based antioxidants.

6. Green leafy vegetables (spinach, kale, chard). Good source of folic acid, which is a B vitamin for the maturation of bone marrow and a preventive for cancer and heart disease.

7. Cruciferous vegetables (broccoli, brussels sprouts, cabbage). Provide glucosinolates, which are sulfur-containing compounds that help the liver detoxify xenobiotics (foreign chemicals).

8. Allium vegetables (onions and garlic). Contain detoxifying sulfur compounds.

9. Flax meal. A good source of omega-3 fatty acids (alpha-linoleic acid), which are generally deficient in the American diet relative to omega-6 fatty acids. The meal is also high in lignans, a type of fiber that is converted into phytoestrogens in the gut, which help to block negative effects of xeno-estrogens like dioxins, which are overstimulating our reproductive systems and predisposing us to breast cancer and infertility.

HEALTHY LIVING WITH DR. MARTIN

ROBERT C. MARTIN, D.C.

"My family and I avoid medical care at almost all costs (drugs, surgery, hospital births, and so on) unless, of course, a life-threatening situation arises or exists," explains Dr. Martin, a chiropractor physician who helps sick people find their way back to health naturally. "Far too many people in the United States opt to utilize medical care and pharmaceuticals for virtually all their maladies and infirmities."

Dr. Martin adds, "I receive hundreds of e-mails weekly, asking for health information and advice. Most of the questions are from people who have either been to their doctor with little or no results or are afraid to see a doctor for fear of what may be found or recommended."

To avoid unnecessary medical care, here are some of the healthy lifestyles that he and his family practice:

- *Drink pure water only.* "Drinking pure water is a way of helping the body to dilute and wash away the impurities we absorb through everyday exposure. Water that's impure, such as tap water, contains many undesirable medications such as chlorine."
- *Forgo beef or pork.* "I grew up on beef and pork. Once I became aware of all the hormones and antibiotics that are fed to the animals, I decided to eliminate them from my family's diet."
- *Stay clear of hydrogenated or partially hydrogenated fats.* "When oils are hydrogenated, certain types of trans fats are formed. Trans fats are those "partially hydrogenated" vegetable oils listed on the labels of so many common foods. Research shows that people who eat more trans fats get more heart attacks. To reduce your exposure to trans fats, you should avoid all fried foods, baked pastry, cookies, cakes, muffins, commercial breads, margarine, and vegetable shortening."
- *Use special air filtration in your home.* "Air quality experts now utilize sophisticated high-tech measuring devices to detect undesirable elements in our air space. In fact, it's been well established that indoor air is less clean than outside air. Using home filtration devices such as electrostatic air filters helps keep unnecessary air pollution to a minimum."
- *Remember, families that play together stay healthy together.* "Our family activities include going on adventures and outings. This might include a mountain hike, walking to the beach, or riding bikes."
- *Get chiropractic spinal checkups.* "The entire family receives regular chiropractic spinal checkups, and care when necessary. This fabulous healing art has been the cornerstone to our family's overall ability to stay healthy naturally."
- *Focus on vegetarian cooking.* "Emphasize on whole grains,

legumes, beans, vegetables, fruits, nuts, and seeds. Additionally, we include the limited use of eggs, fermented dairy, poultry, and cold-water fish."

- *Use supplements when necessary.* "We use vitamins, minerals, herbs, and amino acids for prevention as well as treatment when the need arises."

FIVE BENEFITS OF BREAST FEEDING

"There are so many benefits to both the child and the mother," points out family man Dr. Bob Martin, who believes breast feeding is health insurance for the future as well as the present. Here, he details five benefits:

1. Colostrum, a premilk substance secreted from a mother's breast, is rich in nutrients, calories, water, protein, fat, carbohydrates, and immune-system-stimulating factors.
2. Once a baby begins to receive breast milk, it naturally acquires immunity to many diseases.
3. Breast feeding calms both mother and baby, which aids in bonding as well as nurturing.
4. Also, breast feeding benefits the mother by reducing her risk of breast cancer and provides an important stimulus to her hormone system.
5. Babies who are breast-fed are less likely to develop allergies, asthma, bronchitis, and other upper respiratory infections.

DR. ROYAL'S HOMEOPATHIC METHOD

FLEMMING FULLER ROYAL, M.D.

Remember the film *Erin Brockovich*? Julia Roberts plays a law clerk who discovers a cover-up involving a contaminated local water supply. Well, this is based on a true story. When I spoke with Dr. Flemming Royal, some of his fascinating personal anecdotes seemed all too familiar.

Once a flight surgeon in the Air Force, Dr. Royal is known these days as "the father of homeopathy in Nevada." After practicing general medicine in Eugene, Oregon, he took an alternative route. He became interested in homeopathy (an alternative therapy that works on the premise "Like cures like") and he went to Europe to visit Rinehold Voll, M.D., a well-known German doctor who influenced him greatly. He purchased a device Voll had invented called the Dermatron (which measures very small currents that were believed to be acupuncture meridians) and brought home a suitcase full of homeopathic remedies from Germany that he wanted to test and try in his allergy practice. And he did.

Later, the doctor's daughter became ill. He gave her antibiotics thinking it was a strep infection, but she didn't get better. So he turned to blood testing. A pathologist from the local laboratory called him when he got the test results. He told Dr. Royal that his daughter had leukemia.

Says Dr. Royal, "I quickly brought my daughter to the clinic and tested her with the Dermatron. I discovered that she had been poisoned with pesticides." Later he learned that they came from his house in Eugene, Oregon. "I found that I could neutralize those poisons with some homeopathic medicines that I brought back from Germany. I gave her those medicines and within about two weeks she was completely normal." Today she's married to a chiropractic physician and has three children.

Since then, Dr. Royal has had many more success stories by using the Dermatron and homeopathic remedies to counteract other toxic effects, such as radiation poisoning in himself. After feeling ill for a while, he took the matter into his own hands.

"I started testing everything I could, and what showed up was Clark County water. I have a friend who works in the Clark County Water District and I asked him if he would check to see if there was any radiation in the water supply. He called me the next day and started reading off all these different types of radioactive materials, but he said that they are in such tiny doses they don't cause any problem. I took my radium bromide, which is a homeopathic medicine made from radium, and my symptoms disappeared," explains Dr. Royal.

These days, Dr. Royal, a heroic doctor form of the unforgettable sleuth Erin Brockovich, helps folks to detect toxins such as environmental pollutants and remedy them with homeopathic treatments to achieve good health and wellness.

DR. HAIMES'S DETOXIFYING TREATMENTS

LEONARD HAIMES, M.D.

Dr. Leonard Haimes is another doctor who knows how toxins in our environment can affect the human body. His philosophy is simple: "The detoxification process will occur if we get our body in better balance. And all of the things we will do to put it in better balance will help the system get rid of toxins," he explains.

"Anything that we can do to maximize the function of the individual or the individual cells of the body will put us in a position to avoid disease, have a better a quality of life, and also slow down the aging process," adds Dr. Haimes.

Here are some of the noninvasive treatments Dr. Haimes provides to his patients to find out what the underlying cause of a health problem may be:

- *Electroacupuncture.* Dr. Haimes focuses on body chemistry. To get that as close to perfection as possible, like Dr. Flemming Royal, he'll turn to electrodermal testing—EAV—that's electroacupuncture, he explains. So what exactly does this diagnostic procedure, electroacupuncture, do?

   "It will look at energy flows through the body. It does use the Chinese meridian system, but there are no needles involved. It looks at all of the organs in the body and also down to the cellular level. Actually the instrument works almost like a lie detector. It will ask the body, 'Is this something that you need or don't need?' or 'Is there something we

have to remove?' or 'Is this something you're allergic to?' "
he explains.

- *Homeopathy*. Adds Dr. Haimes, "From the analysis, we come up with a customized homeopathic correction for that individual. Homeopathy is micro dilutions of natural substances. The purpose is to stimulate the body to do its own work more effectively. The best analogy I can give you is this: Let's say you walked into a dark room and flipped on the light switch. What happens? There is a connection to the switch and the message goes up to the wire and the light comes on. In homeopathy what we're doing is flipping on the correct switches in an individual's body so it will start working more effectively."

- *Chelation therapy*. This is an intravenous method of cleaning out plaque in the arteries. It also removes toxic metals such as lead, mercury, and aluminum, which can adversely affect the overall function of the body. So Dr. Haimes's mission is to help detoxify people and then let their bodies function in the most efficient way possible.

"We live in a very polluted environment," concludes Dr. Haimes, "and because of that I think that this is effective for our everyday health and longevity."

THREE WAYS DR. HAIMES DETOXIFIES HIS OWN BODY

1. He avoids refined sugars, white flour products, and caffeine; decreases fats; drinks alcohol in moderation; and limits dairy products (butter, margarine, milk, cheese, and yogurt).
2. He does aerobic exercise to get his heart rate up. "When you exercise you sweat; when you sweat you get rid of toxins."
3. He will occasionally go on a three- to five-day strict fast, taking nothing but water or juice. "I usually do it during the change of seasons."

THE DOC'S SUPPLEMENT LIST

Dr. Haimes takes high-quality supplements (hypoallergenic vitamins with no starch, sugar, or pesticides).

Supplement	What It Does
Multivitamin-and-mineral supplement (without iron)	While a multivitamin ensures getting essential vitamins and minerals for optimal health, Dr. Haimes doesn't need iron because he is not anemic and excessive iron can increase your risk of developing cancer and heart disease
Vitamin C	It is an antioxidant that will negate the effect of free radicals; it's also an anti-stress vitamin
Vitamin E	It is another antioxidant that helps fight disease-causing free radicals
CoQ_{10}	It is another antioxidant that is heart-healthy
Magnesium	It is a mineral that is good to help prevent heart disease
Shark liver oil	It's a powerful immune system builder and counteracts the effects of radiation (from televisions, computers, and so on); one of the essential fatty acids important for overall metabolism
Human growth hormone	It's a powerful anti-aging substance that helps build up the immune system

Safety Smarts: Vitamin C: If you take too much, it can cause gastrointestinal problems.

DR. VICZAY'S PERFECT FOOD

MARIKA VON VICZAY, PH.D., N.D., M.D.

When I asked Dr. Marika von Viczay what supplement has and will keep her healthy until 2020, she simply answered: "Spirulina!" Images of the science fiction movie *Soylent Green,* in which starving people ate synthetic nutritious wafers to survive, came to mind as she told me about her fave superfood.

The doctor has been taking this natural superfood (a blue-green alga) since 1972. And she feels this natural antioxidant, which is believed to fight free radicals, is one of the keys to her good health and longevity.

"It's basically the perfect food," she points out. " Even if you goof up on your diet you get the proper cellular nutrition. It maintains a cellular integrity, which means it provides you with unpolluted, clean, good food. " In other words, if you don't get all the essential nutrients in your daily diet this is going to help you keep your cells healthy. "Absolutely!" she says.

In addition to staying healthy, Dr. Viczay keeps her lymphatic system in good order by Light Emission Therapy (which helps restore and maintain the lymphatic circulation). Web site: www.lymph detox.com.

DOC'S RX TO HEAL YOURSELF

- Consider trying a juice-cleansing diet to detox your body.
- Eat detoxifying superfoods such as fresh fruits and vegetables to stave off toxins.
- Follow a healthful lifestyle—pure water, clean air, more vegetables, and less beef, pork, and hydrogenated fats.
- Supplement your diet with vitamins and minerals for prevention or treatment as needed.
- Opt for detoxifying homeopathic remedies, electroacupunc-

ture, and chelation therapy if you are having health problems.

- Remember to take detoxifying supplements such as antioxidants vitamin C, A, and CoQ_{10} and shark liver oil.
- Consider taking spirulina, which provides you with unpolluted, clean food.

BIOS

Elson M. Haas, M.D., is a family doctor and takes care of people
of all ages with all kinds of problems. He is the founder and medical director of Preventive Medical Center of Marin, California.
He attended the University of Michigan. He is the author of
*Staying Healthy with Nutrition, Staying Healthy with the Sea-
sons,* and *The Detox Diet* (all published by Ten Speed Press). At
53, he lives in Sebastopol, California, with his wife and two children. Web site: www.Elsonhaas.com.

Leonard Haimes, M.D., is a 73-year-old doctor in practice at the
Haimes Centre in Boca Raton, Florida. He received his degree at
Hahnemann Medical College in Philadelphia, Pennsylvania. He is
trained in internal medicine and now practices complementary
medicine. Dr. Haimes is married and has three children.

Robert C. Martin, D.C., is a chiropractic physician, board-certified
clinical nutritionist, board-certified anti-aging doctor, and board-
certified physiotherapist. He attended Palmer College of Chiropractic in Davenport, Iowa. His two web sites are www.drbob
martin.com and www.nutritionaltest.com. He invented the first
nutritional supplement called HearAll. He resides in Scottsdale,
Arizona, with his wife and six children.

Robert Rountree, M.D., is a family physician. He attended medical school at University of North Carolina at Chapel Hill. At 48,
he is in private practice in Boulder, Colorado, where he lives with

his significant other and her two children, a 9-year-old boy and an 11-year-old girl.

Flemming Fuller Royal, M.D., is a holistically oriented physician who graduated from Bourman Gray Medical School in North Carolina. He has a practice, the Nevada Clinic, Integrated Medicine for Health and Wellness, in Las Vegas, Nevada. At 67, he is married, has four children, and lives in Las Vegas.

Marika von Viczay, Ph.D., N.D., M.D., is board certified as a naturopathic physician from Washington, D.C. She received her M.D. degree in Austria and her Ph.D. in psychology at New York University in New York City. At 66, she is a member of the American Academy of Anti-Aging Medicine. She lives in Asheville, North Carolina, and has one daughter and one grandchild.

38

Spirituality and Health

DR. KOENIG'S HEALING POWER OF FAITH

HAROLD G. KOENIG, M.D.

Adele, a senior friend of mine, endured the death of her husband and brother. Her religious activities and belief have eased the emotional pain of these events. Not only does her faith in God give her strength, but it also keeps her in touch with other people. And this spiritual force helps her stay happy and healthy.

Adele's healing power of faith is no surprise to Harold G. Koenig, M.D., a psychiatrist who knows that religious beliefs and practices are associated with greater well-being and life satisfaction, as well as better physical health and longer life. "I help people who have depression, anxiety, those who have problems with their memory," he says. And occasionally he'll bring spirituality to those who are in need.

In other words, there's a sense that somebody is in control when everything seems out of control. "That God cares about the situation. That there is a personal God that is in control, and we can talk to that God and we can do that together," explains Dr. Koenig, a Christian.

Deepening one's personal spirituality can help to close the separateness and isolation that Adele, and other people, can feel during troubled times. "It helps to diminish that, as a connection is made spiritually, in many respects, in this triangle between her and God, me and her, and me and God."

So does Dr. Koenig, author of *The Healing Power of Faith* (Simon & Schuster), use religion and spirituality in his own life? "Yes, I do," he answers. "I've climbed some of the highest mountains in the world, I've been a boxer, and I've been a wrestler. Then I was struck down by a crippling arthritis to cope with for the last 20 years." But faith has played an enormous part in his life, he told me.

"I pray every day. I pray in the morning for about 30 minutes. I read scriptures at night. I also pray about an hour before I go to bed. I pray with my family, my wife and kids. I attend a local church regularly and am involved in that religious community."

But how? How exactly does having a spiritual force in the doctor's life help him to stay balanced? "In many ways," he answers.

- *Mentally.* "It helps me to put things in perspective. When I'm worrying about something, I'll take it into prayer in the morning or evening. That will help me to realize what is important and what is not important. That immediately reduces my stress level."
- *Physically.* "It helps my body because it affects me mentally. The fact that I'm at peace, that I have a sense of purpose in my life, that I can forgive easier, that I can be more outgoing, loving, and caring toward others—all of those things have physiological consequences. My blood pressure is about 110/60 despite the fact that my dad and grandfather both had hypertension.

  "If I pray it makes a huge difference. Otherwise that would make me feel very much out of control, worried about the future. Because of my relationship with God, I know that he is in control and that gives me peace in the situation that I am in."
- *Spiritually.* "When you talk about spirit I think I'm also talk-

ing about my psychological mood, and ability to handle things—sense of peace and purpose and well-being. All of that is enhanced by prayer, but in particular by my relationship with God, which prayer nourishes. I certainly have experienced life more abundantly, and I have seen others experience it more abundantly since they developed a personal relationship with God."

SUCCESS STORY

Sally was a 49-year-old professor who was hit with a tidal wave of emotional woes, from work to relationship problems. Dr. Koenig recalls, "She was frantic, had broken down in my office and was literally hysterical. I asked her if it would help if we said a little prayer. So I said a very short prayer expressing God's love for her, his understanding, and asking for his peace for her. That meant the world to her and completely calmed her down. She was thankful and squeezed my hand." The best part was, she was able to continue her day.

People like Sally often find strength in religion, says Dr. Koenig. "Religion and spirituality were important to her. Having a doctor address that very important part of her life, I think, was very meaningful for her."

DOC'S RX TO HEAL YOURSELF

- Having a spiritual force in your life can provide a feeling of connection.
- Prayer can help you to put life's stresses in perspective.
- Maintaining a relationship with God can help you to stay calm and cope with health problems, from lowering blood pressure to soothing arthritis aches and pains.
- The healing power of faith can help you to have health, peace, and wellness.

Bio

Harold G. Koenig, M.D., is an associate professor of psychiatry and medicine at Durham, North Carolina–based Duke University Medical Center and director of Duke's Center for the Study of Religion/Spirituality and Health; he is the author of *The Healing Power of Faith* (Simon & Schuster) and *Handbook of Religion and Health* (Oxford University Press). He resides in Durham, North Carolina. He is 49, is married, and has two children and three pets.

39

Physician, Heal Thyself

Q & A WITH DR. EDELL

DEAN EDELL, M.D.

Who in the world can you can ring up for one-on-one down-to-earth medical advice? Dr. Dean Edell, of course! He is a hugely popular radio and television doctor (one of the first) whose daily broadcasts are heard by more than 10 million fans each week. Indeed, people of all ages can and do ask personal health questions and Dr. Edell provides straightforward answers.

Now the doctor, a former general surgeon and eye surgeon, who became a media doctor when opportunity knocked, has been put to the test. One day in a telephone interview he answered personal questions from his home office. It was an unique experience to be able to hear what this energetic doctor's health regimen is. After all, I have been listening to him for years on the radio and TV as he's helped countless people. And now, this celebrity doctor was ready to tell me how *he* enjoys life and stays health.

Q. *Why do you feel America is becoming so obsessed with health?*
A. Life is so good in America. But with the media constantly telling us about all the dangers and the scary things out there, we have now become anxiety-ridden and we obsess about it. It doesn't make sense. It's almost like an attitude that's developed. So we have these fears. At the same time, we're living longer than we ever have. Heart disease rates continue to plummet. Cancer the same. And yet we all perceive ourselves as being less healthy. We're afraid to eat the food, drink the water, or breath the air. We're told that we're nothing but a bunch of fat, lazy slobs. And a huge medical-health complex has grown up to constantly keep us anxiety-ridden so we'll take their pills, take their tests, and jump through the hoops.

Q. *You say you've been blessed with great genes. Does that mean if our parents are healthy the odds are that we'll be healthy, too?*
A. Absolutely. The single most important factor in determining your own longevity is the longevity of your parents—more than the amount of exercise and cholesterol levels. But you can't count on it. You can't count on anything. So you've got to sit down and look at all those factors and how they add up. If you have a brother or sister who has lived to be 100, that is the single most significant boost of longevity anyone on earth could have. It seems that siblings can be more important because parents are genetically more different than your sibling.

Q. *You say that in America if everyone ate a 30 percent fat diet, the average male would live four months longer. But then you add that most people would hate eating like that—it might not be worth it. Why not?*
A. Well, because if you get four months extra in the nursing home it might not be worth all that effort. First, 30 percent of the people who eat that diet are going to be made worse by it, 30 percent will see no change, and 30 percent will have some advantage. If you don't know who you are ahead of time, over millions and millions of people that adds up to a significant health issue. But if you can't stand eating a low-fat diet then you're nuts to do it all

your life when there are other things you can do that will have even more of an effect.

Q. *Other things?*
A. Sex has more of an effect. Exercise may or may not. Having social relationships and friends. Having a glass of wine a day has more of an effect than that of a low-fat diet.

Q. *You personally eat a lower-saturated-fat diet at home but you pig out at restaurants. What is the message here?*
A. Moderation is the key. Anything more extreme you ought to do because you really enjoy it and you just want to do it. But you're kidding yourself if you think you're getting some automatic pass to health nirvana. Because it isn't going to happen that way, unfortunately. We just don't know for the individual what these effects would be. So when you exercise it doesn't take more than an hour or two a week of walking to get almost the maximum benefit of exercise. And many people do too much. There's a lot of folks out there who become obsessive about it. America would be better off if everybody got up and took a walk for half an hour once a week than all the people clogging the gyms right now. But that's not happening.

Q. *So you told me that you personally don't exercise but you do stay active by shopping or carrying firewood. Explain how this keeps you healthy.*
A. I'm a high-energy person. I hate exercise. I can't think of anything more boring. I like doing things. I'm about 6'4" and 180 pounds and I've been that since college. And I don't lift a finger in terms of exercise. My father is the same way. He's 88 years old, and he weighs about the same as I do. And he's eaten meat loaf all of his life and never has exercised either.

Q. *Do you think it's important to eat a well-balanced nutrient-dense diet?*
A. Absolutely. The most important thing that people have got to realize is that now that we've learned more about this, there are more of these micronutrients and vitamins that you do not get in pills that are contained in vegetables and fruits. We've discovered

lycopene in tomatoes and all kinds of things that are important to your health.

Q. *What do you personally do to unwind for your health's sake?*
A. I get out of town. It's the only way I can do it. Can't do it around here. I can get away from the phones, the kids, household chores, and all the things that are enough to drive anyone off the edge of the earth. I'll drive up to the middle of northern California's redwood forest and just stay there for a few days. I come back and feel like a stranger in a strange land. It's a matter of focusing your brain on something other than the craziness that we all deal with. And that balance seems to be associated with longevity. And there's been lots and lots of studies now on this mind-body effect.

Q. *You seem to be saying, live life, be happy. Is that really the route to good health and longevity?*
A. I have no doubt. Ask yourself the following question: "Are you better off living well but shorter, or longer and being miserable?" Even if that were the choice, which I don't think it is, there is a case to be made for enjoying life. We are *not* all guaranteed to live the same length of time and get the same diseases. So it's like people who save, save, save money every day and don't spend money and have fun with it thinking sometime at the end of their life they're going to get a chance to enjoy it. And then you'll see them drop dead at 60. And all of sudden you think, "Oh my gosh, there are no guarantees." Build in the joy now as much as you can.

DOC'S RX TO HEAL YOURSELF

- Genes count when it comes to longevity.
- Enjoy the good things in life—lovemaking, social relationships, and even a glass of wine—which can enhance good health.
- Practice moderation in your diet.
- Stay physically active.

- Eat a nutrient-dense diet including plenty of fruits and vegetables, which can keep you healthy.
- Learn how to deplug from a hectic twenty-first-century lifestyle to calm your mind and body.
- Live life and be happy.

BIO

Dean Edell, M.D., is a popular radio and television personality, at 60, who broadcasts nationally on TV and radio. A graduate of Cornell University Medical College, he lives in the San Francisco Bay Area. He is the author of *Eat, Drink and Be Merry* (Quill, an imprint of HarperCollins Publishers). "We have eight children between us. I have five kids that are truly products of my loins and three stepchildren." Web site: HealthCentral.com.

40

Future Health

OH BABY! WITH DR. BREWER

SARAH BREWER, M.D.

These days, women are a lot more on top of matters of prenatal care than our moms were. Dr. Sarah Brewer is just one of those baby-smart women who know just what to do to keep it safe the full nine months. Take a look at what the doctor did while she was pregnant.

- *Avoid alcohol.* "I avoided alcohol for three months before conception and for the nine months of pregnancy. I stayed clear of wine for at least a year (a real sacrifice, as I've studied for my wine diploma exams and really enjoy wine tastings)."
- *Team Up.* "I put my partner on a preconceptual sperm-boosting program: no alcohol. (I got him to stop smoking before conceiving the first time around.) Boxer shorts, anti-oxidant supplements including vitamins C and E, carotenoids, selenium, and zinc. These measures have all been shown to boost the quality and quantity of sperm. Must have worked, as we went on to conceive twins!"

- *Do easy exercise.* "Gentle exercise program with my partner: jogging one or two miles three times a week for six
  months to get fit for pregnancy. At the age of 40, pregnancy
  can be grueling. This time around I felt much fitter than four
  years previously as a result, with no swollen ankles and very
  little tiredness despite carrying twins."
- *Play supplement switcheroo.* "I changed to a folic acid–containing multivitamin-and-mineral supplement designed for
  pregnancy a month before stopping contraception, to reduce
  the risk of developmental defects."
- *Take more primrose oil.* "I increased evening primrose oil to
  2 grams daily. Anecdotal evidence suggests it prevents
  stretch marks. Despite my having a 54-inch waist at the end,
  not a single stretch mark in sight!"
- *Add fish oil.* "I started eating more oily fish (salmon), and
  started fish oil supplements designed for pregnancy. These
  essential fatty acid supplements boost development of the
  baby's eyes and brain."
- *Use Baby Plus.* "At 24 weeks I started a prenatal stimulation
  program using Baby Plus (a unit that you clip to your waist-
  band and which plays a series of repetitive sounds similar to
  the heartbeat, which, over 16 weeks, become increasingly
  rapid to stimulate the baby's hearing and brains cells)."
  [http://www.babyplus.com]
- *Practice meditation.* "I meditated once a day where possible
  for relaxation."
- *Pamper yourself.* "I had daily massage from my partner,
  rubbing in Beautiful Belly Balm (a rich moisturizing oint-
  ment designed to help the skin stretch) on my abdomen and
  evening primrose oil moisturizer elsewhere to improve skin
  suppleness. My partner also painted my toenails regularly—
  you need to feel thoroughly pampered when you are pregnant!" [To order Beautiful Belly Balm and fish oil supplement
  designed for pregnancy log onto www.pregnancy-shop.com]
- *Breast-feed.* "I breast-fed for four months as this is the time
  shown to give optimum benefits for immunity and brain development. I would have liked to continue to nine months as

I did with my first child, but feeding twins and writing full-time was too exhausting so I had to stop."

THE DOC'S SUPPLEMENT LIST

Here is Dr. Brewer's personal list for supplements when she was pregnant.

Supplement	What It Does
Multivitamin-and-mineral supplement	Folic acid–containing supplement to reduce risk of developmental defects
Primrose oil	A supplement that prevents stretch marks
Fish oils	Essential fatty acids help boost development of baby's eyes and brain

Safety Smarts: Omega-3 oils: Don't take high doses of fish oil capsules if you are taking NSAIDs (nonsteroidal anti-inflammatory drugs). It may increase gastrointestinal ulcers and bleeding.

DR. PESCATORE TEACHES OUR CHILDREN WELL

FRED PESCATORE, M.D.

As an internist, Fred Pescatore, M.D., and author of *Feed Your Kids Well* (John Wiley & Sons) *gets it* about healthy eating for children, perhaps because he was overweight when he was a child. "My big interest is to have no other child go through what I went through," he told me. He wants parents to get it, too, so they can prevent the emotional and physical torment overweight kids may experience if they tilt the scales.

These days, Dr. Pescatore is lean and has his weight under control. Here are his solutions to common problems of kids and what they eat.

Too much sugar, soda, and fruit juice. The biggest issue that most children have with sugar is that they don't realize what it is doing to them in the long run. Studies show that it makes them overweight. One in three kids in this country are overweight. Children who drink one extra soda a day have a 65 percent chance of becoming overweight. And so if they're not in the habit of drinking soda and fruit juice, they'll never be in the habit.

Healthy Eating Solution. Drink flavored seltzers, which taste just like sodas. Or drink more water. The amount goes by weight. (If they're 40 pounds they should be drinking 25 ounces; if 80 pounds they should be drinking 40 ounces. It's divisible by 2.)

Unhealthy eating habits. Habits are formed when children are young. Healthy eating should be as important a habit as brushing your teeth, combing your hair, doing well in school, and having polite manners.

Healthy Eating Solution. "Train and teach our kids what healthy eating is right from the beginning. All too often we allow our kids to take control of what food they eat at a very early age. If we take a little bit of the control back around food and around healthy eating, they'll learn how to respect that," he says. Remember how Mom dished up comfort food—ice cream, cake—when you weren't feeling well? That comfort turns into an unhealthy eating habit. It's best to learn proper eating habits when we're young.

Eating too much. Blame it on the lifestyle that we have created. Television and Internet commercials put us smack into a food culture. "And we have children who don't know how to process that information," says Dr. Pescatore. "They're eating too many fast foods, too many of the processed foods and sugar. It becomes a real big health issue because we have a sixfold increase in diabetes in children."

Healthy Eating Solution. How do we get our kids away from the processed, microwave stuff and eat real fresh food? "We have to teach them what is healthy and what is not healthy. You have to introduce a child to a new food 20 to 25 times before they're going to eat it. It's not just enough to give it to them once or twice and say, "Oh, my son or daughter doesn't like that," says Dr. Pescatore. Plus, you have to be a good role model and eat healthy foods to set a healthy example for your kids.

Not enough exercise. Sadly enough, some schools have had their physical education programs cut for budgetary reasons. In most states now it's not mandatory, and that leads to sofa spud kids.

Healthy Eating Solution. Best advice: Increase lifestyle activities. "I'm not telling you to go out and join the gym and buy all this equipment," says Dr. Pescatore. "Instead, he suggests a family outing such as bowling."

Poor lifestyle. Latchkey kids are tempted to eat unhealthful, convenient fast food or junk food. Plus, when teens are unsupervised, they may find cigarettes, alcohol, or drugs alluring.

Healthy Eating Solution. More family interaction can promote healthful living. Instead of going to the mall and everybody scurrying to find the closest parking spot they can, park at the farthest spot and walk. Take your child to the grocery store because there they can not only learn about food, they can also push the grocery cart of these big supermarkets that we have now.

Q & A WITH DR. ULLIS

KARLIS ULLIS, M.D.

Q. *Why do you feel baby boomers [the 76 million Americans born between 1946 and 1964] are so obsessed with aging in America?*

A. They are obsessed about losing control of their appearance. They've seen their parents. Just go to Eastern Europe and see what a 50-year-old looks like. They are acting like a 1950s generation—red meat and cigarettes.

Q. *I am a baby boomer, and I am so much healthier than my mother was. I'm not alone, right?*
A. Baby boomers who are in their forties, like you, have been following Adele Davis since age 15. So there are anti-aging patients of mine who have been brought up on raw, natural food, and you can see the difference.

Q. *In my teens I rebelled against my mother's meat-and-potatoes type of diet. Is that unheard of?*
A. No, it was part of that rebellion. That's what makes the baby boomers who they are. They are rebellious of getting old. They are post-hippies. They cut their hair, they've become established, but they're not going to lie down, roll over, and play dead.

Q. *What about the X-generation? I've been hearing from some of the 101 doctors that Generation X is not as health-conscious as the baby boomers?*
A. The Generation X is defined as between 20 and 30. They're worried, they're anxious. They didn't play like we did. I went to UCLA, and there are no dogs and frisbees on campus anymore. I think people who grew up in the 1960s somehow are connected by the aging boomer thing. Because in the 1960s there was a certain purity of Hinduism, your soul, your inner self. There is a little of that element left. There is still a remnant of that left over, but you don't see it in the Generation X-ers, because they never went through that.

Q. *Is the key to go back to nature like the baby boomers did and are doing?*
A. I have an e-mail group of anti-aging patients called "39 Forever." It's really interesting: When one patient says she can't sleep because of her menopausal transition, everybody is really supportive. Andropause, menopause—I see it every day.

Q. *Yeah, but baby boomers are taking the healthy route, whereas our moms and dads did not, right?*
A. There are a lot of natural alternatives. Women can take a lot of natural herbs and other things where you don't have to go on a lot of hormones.

Q. *So what's the deal? Are the baby boomers on the right anti-aging track?*
A. The post-hippie generation has a spark of enlightenment that Generation X does not have. I think there is a spark of enlightenment in these individuals that I see, like yourself, and the people I talk to in this age group, who are just a little bit more enlightened. Generation X is in the dark.

Q. *Although you're not a baby boomer, what's your personal anti-aging plan?*
A. I was on human growth hormone injections for a year and a half. I decided that this was garbage and I was going to go low-tech—natural. Caloric restriction. The most evidence we have on aging systems goes back to caloric restrictions of animals—birds, fish, and other species. I'm cutting down on calories but I'm eating well.

Q. *What about nutrients?*
A. I take a lot of nutrients. I do not get enough vitamin E in my diet. I don't get enough CoQ_{10}. I don't get enough alpha-lipoic acid. I don't get enough of the Bs. So I take supplements. I know where vitamin E comes from—either soybeans or wheat germ—and I'm not eating enough to get enough vitamin E. CoQ_{10} comes from meat, and I'm not eating enough raw beef heart or liver to get CoQ_{10}.

Q. *Exercise?*
A. Weight training twice a week. Cardiovascular about three to four times a week. And then stretching and yoga.

Q. *The bulk of these 101 doctors are very dedicated to diet, supplements, and exercise—like you—a pre–baby boomer. It's all so anti-aging. But who would want to live to 100?*

A. I would! There's a lot of things I want to see and do. I know what's going on in aging research and in 15 years we're going to have amazing things come our way. It's going to be profound what you're going to have available. You're going to have an extended lifespan and an extended healthspan.

Q. *Do you promise?*
A. I promise!

THE DOC'S SUPPLEMENT LIST

Here are the forever-young supplements that Dr. Ullis recommends.

Supplement	What It Does
CoQ_{10}	A fat-soluble antioxidant that can help prevent heart disease
B vitamins	Helps to lower homocysteine, the amino acid, which can help stave off heart disease
Alpha-lipoic acid	A heart-healthy antioxidant that is good for your arteries
Vitamin E	Antioxidant that helps the immune response especially as we age

Safety Smarts: If you are diabetic and taking insulin, lipoic acid can lower your blood glucose level, which may lower your need for medications. Talk to your doctor.

65 PLUS WITH DR. HARRIS'S GOLDEN RULES

STEVEN HARRIS, M.D.

While the graying of America continues, Dr. Steven Harris, a baby boomer, has a genuine special interest in seniors. Aging experts believe people over 65 will comprise at least 20 percent of the population by the year 2025. And since there is a graying population, there will be a greater awareness and acceptance of aging.

Dr. Harris believes that if we follow these golden rules before our golden years (as he does), we'll live healthier and longer lives before and after we hit age 65.

- *Learn how to take your own vital signs.* That means your pulse, temperature, blood pressure, and your breathing rate are what's going to tell you whether you have a problem that requires a hospital visit or a doctor's appointment. For instance, a high temperature means nothing when you are a child, but it is more likely to be life-threatening illness when you're over 65, explains Dr. Harris.
- *Do whatever it takes to control your blood pressure, cholesterol, and weight.* "If your numbers are high and diet, supplements, and lifestyle changes aren't helping," says Dr. Harris, "do whatever it takes to get those numbers down to prevent a life-threatening disease such as a stroke."
- *Take a good multivitamin-and-mineral supplement.* This will help you get your daily nutrients, which will help prevent disease.
- *Get exercise every day.* Physical activity, such as walking at least 20 minutes daily, will make you stronger and less likely to fall down and break a bone, which is a major cause of disability, particularly in elderly women.
- *Get regular tests.* Women have to know their bone density and get their mammograms; men have to see a urologist regularly.

- *Get a colonoscopy regularly.* If your health plan doesn't pay for it, pay for it yourself to make sure you don't have polyps, which can turn into colon cancer.
- *If you have any cardiovascular risk, consider taking aspirin.* Take one baby aspirin a day (it's not as hard on your stomach).
- *Subscribe to a health magazine and read it.* This will help you to stay up-to-date on preventive health care.

THE DOC'S SUPPLEMENT LIST

Here are the important supplements Dr. Harris recommends.

Supplement	What It Does
Folic Acid	This B vitamin can help lower the homocysteine level in your body and protect against heart disease
Selenium	This antioxidant trace mineral can help you lower your risk of developing cancers

Safety Smarts: Selenium: Too much (more than 600 mcg per day) can be harmful.

DR. HUEMER'S SECRET TO BLISS

RICHARD P. HUEMER, M.D.

Dr. Richard Huemer provides his own words of wisdom on finding good health and happiness:

Jonathan Swift said it, three centuries ago: "The best doctors in the world are Doctor Diet, Doctor Quiet, and Doctor Merryman." They are actually the assistant doctors to the greatest physician of all, the Doctor Within. That is my name for the body's innate ability to heal itself when given the tools to do so.

Doctor Diet is first. We need to get back to the whole, natural foods with as little processing and preparation as possible. We need to scrap that ubiquitous food pyramid, which, like the pyramids in ancient lands, supports superstitious beliefs—in this case, the faith that the pyramid actually has anything to do with good nutrition.

Let's build a new food pyramid with a broad base of fresh vegetables and fruits, with plenty of room for fiber and beneficial fats from fish, legumes, and seeds, and no space at all for refined carbohydrates, trans fats, and food additives. Let's further nourish and protect our bodies with supplemental micronutrients and phytochemicals, which, for the first time in human history, science has made available to us.

As for Doctor Quiet and Doctor Merryman, they are increasingly elusive in modern times, but well worth pursuing as the spiritual side of healing. The science of pyschoneuroimmunology testifies to their central importance in health.

For me personally, they were always harder to relate to than nutritional biochemistry. One day, when I was facing a difficult decision, a patient gave me a bit of advice that made everything clear. She said simply, "Dr. Huemer, follow your bliss." I tell others to do likewise.

DOC'S RX TO HEAL YOURSELF

- To keep our future generation healthy, include a multivitamin-and-mineral and fish oil in your healthy prenatal program.
- Feed your kids and teenagers healthy foods and provide physical activities.
- Eat right—shun unhealthy or simple carbs, trans fats, and additives.
- Accept aging gracefully and go natural without polluting your body, mind, or soul.

- Take anti-aging supplements—vitamin E, alpha-lipoic acid, the B vitamins, CoQ_{10}—to stall the aging process.
- Learn how to take your own vitals and control your blood pressure, cholesterol, and weight A.S.A.P.
- Exercise regularly and stay active.
- Get a physical checkup as part of your preventive health plan to stay healthy physically, mentally, and spiritually.

BIOS

Sarah Brewer, M.D., is a 42-year-old doctor who works in genitourinary medicine and sexual health. She attended Selwyn College, Cambridge, and Cambridge Clinical School. She has written numerous health-related books such as *Planning a Baby?* (Crown) and *Super Baby* (Thorson's). She lives in Norfolk, England, with her husband and three children. Web site: www.medi lance.com.

Steven Harris, M.D., is board certified in internal medicine and geriatrics. He received his medical degree at the University of Utah School of Medicine. He is a 44-year-old medical researcher. He resides in Salt Lake City, Utah.

Richard P. Huemer, M.D., graduated from UCLA School of Medicine in 1958. His background includes basic biomedical research in aging and cancer immunology. He has practiced nutritional and orthomolecular medicine since 1975. He is a longtime health columnist for *Let's Live Magazine,* and the coauthor of *The Natural Health Guide to Beating the Supergerms* (Pocket Books). At 68, he is semi-retired and lives in Palmdale, California, with his wife.

Fred Pescatore, M.D., is an internist and director of the Center of Integrative Medicine in New York. He is the author of *Feed Your Kids Well* (John Wiley & Sons) and *Thin for Good* (John Wiley

& Sons). At 38, he is married and lives in New York City. Web site: www.viplenish.

Karlis Ullis, M.D., specializes in sports medicine and anti-aging. He received his M.D. at the University of Washington in Seattle. He is a 56-year-old assistant clinical professor at UCLA School of Medicine, Los Angeles, California, and medical director at the Sports Medicine and Anti-Aging Medical Group. He has two daughters and lives in Pacific Palisades, California. Web site: www. AgingPrevent.com.

A Final Word

Are you inspired by the preventive strategies that the 101 doctors in this book use for themselves, family, and patients to stay healthy year-round? Here are some guidelines to put you on the doctors' track for life:

- Eat a nutrient-dense diet chock-full of fresh fruits, vegetables, and whole grains.
- Avoid processed foods, sugar, and empty-calorie snacks.
- Include vitamins, minerals, and herbs to supplement your diet as needed to ensure you're getting adequate nutrition every day and to help prevent illness.
- Get preventive physical checkups to maintain your body and well-being.
- Exercise regularly to keep your body functioning at its optimum best.
- Learn how to chill out and enjoy living a longer and healthier life.
- Nourish your body, mind, and spirit each and every day.

As you can see, the 101 doctors in this book have learned how to incorporate lifestyle changes into their diet and exercise plan. These inspirational men and women who face disease and aging, like you and me, practice what they preach. They practice preventive health.

The 101 doctors are role models who have inspired me to be a healthier person. While discussing their personal programs day after day, I couldn't help being touched by their miraculous efforts and devotion to staying healthy.

You too can put lifestyle changes to work in your own life. When you incorporate some of the 101 doctors' diet, supplement, and lifestyle changes into your daily regime, you will gain a new and improved body, mind, and spirit. You can count on it.

For More Information

Following are telephone numbers and website addresses to get more information on products mentioned in this book.

Baby Plus
Website: *www.babyplus.com*

Botox
Phone: 800-44BOTOX or 800-530-6680

The Holistic Dental Digest Plus, a bi-monthly newsletter
Phone: 212-874-4212

LearnTM
Phone: 888-LEARNTM

Migra-Lieve
Phone: 800-758-8746

The Natural Dentist Herbal Mouth and Gum Therapy
Phone: 800-615-6895

Worry Free™
Phone: 800-255-8332
Website: *www.mapi.com*

Young Living Essential Oils
Phone: 800-763-9963

Publisher's Resource List

There are over one hundred physicians in this book who are using various supplements for theirs and their families health. The one thing most doctors seem to agree upon is the purchasing of supplements from reliable sources. There are many products available in outlet stores, discount stores and bargain shops. It is virtually impossible to determine if the quality of these brands is totally effective or even safe. We suggest obtaining supplements from health food stores and top ranked mail order houses.

There are many fine supplement houses who manufacture safe, reliable and effective product lines. These companies use only the finest ingredients and have adopted top-quality controls in their manufacturing process. You will find their products in both health food stores and mail order companies. You will find virtually all of the supplements mentioned in this book at the firms listed below. They are among the very best and are recommended by top physicians.

Carlson® Laboratories
1-800-323-4141
www.carlsonlabs.com

Jarrow Formulas™
1-800-726-0886
www.jarrow.com

NutriCology, Inc.
1-800-545-9960
www.nutricology.com

Solgar® Vitamin and Herb
1-800-645-2246
www.solgar.com

Source Naturals®
1-800-815-2333
www.sourcenaturals.com

Twin Lab
1-800-645-5626
www.twinlab.com

Here are some examples of first rate mail order houses:

N.E.E.D.S
1-800-634-1380
www.needs.com
This organization stocks quality supplements from every important manufacturer. Call them for a catalog or check their web site. They also carry a variety of many other products, including environmental.

Wilner Chemists
1-800-633-1106
www.wilner.com
They are the oldest and largest nutritionally oriented pharmacy in the United States. They offer a large selection of nutritional, herbal and homeopathic supplements. Catalog available, or check their web site. This pharmacy is one of the very few who

will do special compounding of special medications that your doctor may require.

Carotec, Inc.
1-800-522-4279
www.carotec.com
This company manufactures their own privately branded line of supplements. All of their products are made with superior and safe ingredients, and many of the products are manufactured to pharmaceutical standards. They have an interesting catalogue that explains how each of their supplements are made and what ingredients they use.

There are firms who specialize in distributing supplements to offices of M.D.'s homeopaths, N.D.'s, chiropractors and other health professionals. Here is one of the finest:

Moss Nutrition
1-800-851-5444
www.mossnutrition.com
This organization supplies quality nutritional supplements exclusively to health care professionals throughout the United States. Having been in existence for ten years, Moss Nutrition has developed contacts with many quality health practitioners of various types throughout the country. If you would like the name of a practitioner in your area who can serve your needs and provide you with these quality supplements, please feel free to call them at the above number.

Just as with regular supplements, it is important that herbs be purchased from only those companies who take pride and care in the way they grow and manufacture their herbal compounds. There are a number of very good herbal companies, but because of space limitation we will list only a few of the very best. The following companies are among the very few that check every batch of herbs for impurities and inferior parts of the plant. These fine products are available in your local health food store.

You can also contact the companies and ask for a store near you that distributes their products.

Herbs

Eclectic Institute, Inc.
1-800-332-4372
www.eclecticherb.com
   Eclectic Institute has developed a line of encapsulated botanicals, which are fresh, freeze-dried instead of air-dried. Why fresh freeze-dried herbs instead of air-dried herbs? Fresh freeze-drying the herbs maintains the active constituents of the natural potency of most herbs. Fresh freeze-drying preserves all of the biologically active constituents of the fresh plant—not just some of the active constituents.

Gaia Herbs
1-800-831-7780
www.gaiaherbs.com
   Founded by Ric Scalzo, Gaia uses mostly certified organic and ecologically wildcrafted herbs that are specifically selected and formulated to work synergistically within the body. This company also has a full line of herbs in capsules and liquid phyto-caps—a revolutionary new delivery system for liquid herbal extracts. All phyto-caps are vegetable-based and alcohol-free.

Herbalist and Alchemist
1-800-611-8235
www.herbalist-alchemist.com
   H & A was founded by herbalist David Winston, A.H.G., and provides some of the highest-quality herbal tinctures and herbal products available in the United States. They have over three hundred herbal products formulated in tinctures. Their formulated tinctures and herbs are mostly organic or wildcrafted. They also have audiotapes available for information about how to use herbs correctly for various body functions.

Planetary Formulas
1-800-606-6226
www.planetherbs.com
   Planetary Formulas makes numerous products combining Western, Chinese, and Ayurvedic herbs. Dr. Michael Tierra, O.M.D., L.Ac., is one of the foremost authorities on herbal medicine in North America and has had a clinical practice for thirty years. He is the product formulator for Planetary Formulas and is an internationally recognized authority on the world's herbal traditions. Planetary Formulas carries a wide range of herbs and herbal formulas in tablets and tinctures extracted with alcohol. They also carry a line of herbs for children with glycerin added to neutralize any alcohol taste.

Organic Culinary Herbs
   An assortment of certified organic culinary herbs that are non-irradiated, unfumigated and packed in glass spice jars, including basil leaves, bay leaves, cayenne pepper, garlic powder, ginger root, turmeric root and many others. Available from:

Natural Lifestyle.
1-800-752-2775
www.natural-lifestyle.com

Liquid Spice Concentrates (liquid culinary herbs)
Cinnamon, Ginger, Chamomile, Lemongrass, Peppermint, Sweet Chai. Each in 1.76 oz. containers. Available from:

Omega Nutrition
1-800-661-3529
www.omeganutrition.com

Mail Order for Herbs

N.E.E.D.S.
1-800-634-1380
www.needs.com

Wilner Chemists
1-800-522-4279
www.wilner.com

If you can't find the herbal supplement you are looking for in your local health food store, try calling N.E.E.D.S. or Wilner Chemists. They carry virtually all of the top herbal lines and will supply a catalog upon request. Both of these organizations always make sure that the products they carry are fresh.

Herbal Advice

If you require the services of a master herbalist for herbal advice relating to any of the medical conditions listed in this book, these people are knowledgeable in Western, Chinese and Ayurvedic herbal modalities.

Chrysalis Natural Medicine Clinic
Alan Keith Tillotson, Ph.D., A.H.G.—Medical Herbalist
Nai-shing Hu Tillotson, O.M.D., L.Ac.—Chinese Medicine
1008 Milltown Road, Wilmington, DE 19808 USA
Phone: 302-994-0565 Fax: 302-995-0653
Email: AlanT3@aol.com

The Chrysalis Natural medicine clinic is highly trained in prescribing herbal medicine treatments for serious or difficult to treat diseases. Phone consultations or office visits are available. Chrysalis maintains a large pharmacy of over 1,000 herbal medicines and nutrients available by mail to any location in the world.

In this special resource section, we have selected foods, teas and oils, which are mostly organic and of the highest quality. Many of the doctors writing within the pages of this book recommend specific foods and teas for good health. This is equally as important as taking the right supplements. Listed are some of the products and organizations that have the highest quality products most of which is organic and are used by many physicians.

Organic Food

Flaxseeds

Living Tree Community Foods
1-800-260-5534
www.livingtreecommunity.com
Organic Golden Flax
　Golden flaxseeds are larger and softer than the dark brown flaxseed. They have a mild nutty flavor that is really delicious mixed in food. This flaxseed has about 31/2 times as much Omega-3 fatty acids as Omega-6 fatty acids. It is also the richest known source of potassium, magnesium, and boron. To maintain a fresh supply grind daily in a coffee grinder.

Omega Nutrition
1-800-661-3529
www.omeganutrition.com
Flax Of Life—Cold Milled Organic Flaxseeds
　Certified-organic flaxseeds, vacuum-packed in a lined, resealable foil bag to retain freshness. Flaxseed is a terrific source of the essential oil Omega 3.

Flax Of Life—Whole Organic Flaxseeds
Certified-organic flaxseeds

Beans

Organic Beans
Dried organic beans
　There are a wide variety available including Aduki domestic,

Blackeye Peas, Black Turtle, Chick Peas, Kidney Beans, Pinto Beans, Navy Beans, Mug Beans, Lentils Green, Lentils Red, Peas Split, Limas Baby. Available from:

Natural Lifestyle
1-800-752-2775
www.natural-lifestyle.com

Teas (Green)

Try switching from coffee to green tea and enjoy the benefits of antioxidants and less caffeine. There is an amino acid in green tea (Camellia sinensis) that balances caffeine's effects and delivers a sense of relaxation.

Maitake Products, Inc.
1-800-747-7418
www.maitake.com
Mai Green™Tea
Contains organically grown maitake mushroom and premier Japanese green tea (matcha) leaves. Low in caffeine. Available in tea bags.

Rishi Tea
866-747-4483 (866-**RISHI TEA**)
www.rishi-tea.com
Rishi imports premium loose-leaf teas directly from tea gardens in Asia. An integral component of tea quality is its purity. Rishi offers more than two dozen certified organic teas, including ten green tea varietals. The positive health benefits of regular consumption of green tea are now well documented and this company sells only high quality loose tea. Usually this will deliver a more potent and healthful drink, as compared to tea packed in tea bags.

Rooibos Tea
Rooibos is an herb that has been used in South Africa for cen-

turies and has been shown to have very high levels of vitamins, minerals and anti-aging properties. Rooibos has a mildly sweet flavor and earthy aroma, as well as some potential health benefits. It contains calcium, iron, zinc, vitamin C and several other important minerals. Rooibos is naturally caffeine free and is believed to relieve insomnia, cramps, constipation, skin irritations and allergic symptoms. Recent research has also shown that it has higher antioxidant concentrations than green tea and contains the highest levels of anti-aging properties of any plant on earth. This is organically grown and in loose-leaf form. Available from **Rishi Tea**

Rooibos Tea is also available in tea bags and is organic. From **Wisdom of the Ancients®** 1-800-899-9908 *www.wisdomherbs.com*

Pu-erh Tea

Even less known, but certainly worthy of investigation is Pu-erh tea. Pu-erh imparts a warming energy and is believed to cleanse the blood and tonify the body. More than any other tea in China, Pu-erh is prized for its medicinal properties.

Available from Rishi Tea

Negata Green Sencha Tea

Nagata organic Japanese green tea is made from the season's first young leaves, hand harvested at their peak of flavor, steamed and dried—mildly stimulating. Green Sencha is available in both bulk tea and in Sencha Haiku tea bags.

Available from **Natural Lifestyle** 1-800-752-2775 *www.natural-lifestyle.com*

Tea Filter Bags from **Rishi Tea**

Loose tea suffers from a stigma of being too complicated to prepare. In fact, loose tea is about as simple as it gets: pouring hot water on tea leaves. Standard tea bags are easy enough, but quality and flavor are sometimes sacrificed.

The main sticking point for many people when brewing loose

tea is having some sort of implement with which to infuse the tea. Teapots are ideal, but if you want something even more convenient, check out the tea filter bags that Rishi Tea uses. It's simple—you spoon the tea leaves into the bag, place the bag in the cup and pour the water on it. In effect, you make your own tea bag. The filter bags are made of all-natural biodegradable hemp fiber and are designed to let the tea leaves expand. Tea balls and clamps, on the other hand, prevent the tea leaves from steeping properly and can introduce heavy metals into tea. A wonderful way to brew loose tea.

Tea Press

Another unique and very easy to use tea press produces a rich full-bodied tea made with a heat resistant tempered glass carafe and a permanent stainless steel filter.

Available from:

Natural Lifestyle
1-800-752-2775
www.natural-lifestyle.com

Triple Leaf Tea, Inc.
1-800-552-7448 *www.tripleleaf-tea.com*
maryanne@tripleleaf-tea.com

Effective, authentic, traditional Chinese green, naturally decaffeinated green, medicinal and diet teas, made with authentic Chinese herbs and traditional herbal formulas, packaged in convenient tea bag form. All teas are GMO-free.

Triple Leaf Tea's Decaf Green Tea and Decaf Green Tea blends uses a natural solvent-free carbon dioxide decaffeination process that researchers have found maintains almost all of green tea's beneficial antioxidants, including EGCG, while leaving no chemical residue. Other decaffeination methods use either a chemical solvent, ethyl acetate, which researchers have found to remove much of the antioxidants, or water, which also is likely to deplete the antioxidants, since they are extremely water-soluble.

If you drink a lot of green tea and don't want the caffeine this is the ideal tea to use.

Decaf Green Tea with Ginseng:
Naturally decaffeinated green tea leaves, honeysuckle flower, chrysanthemum flower, dandelion root, mulberry leaf, peppermint leaf, astragalus root, Siberian ginseng root (Eleutherococcus senticosus), American ginseng root (Panax quinquefolius), Asian ginseng root (Panax ginseng), jiaogulan (Gynostemma pentaphyllum), licorice root.

Ginkgo & Decaf Green Tea:
Ginkgo biloba leaf, naturally decaffeinated green tea leaves, eucommia leaf, Ho Shou Wu (fo ti) root, Poria cocos mushroom, astragalus root, Siberian ginseng root (Eleutherococcus senticosus), American ginseng root (Panax quinquefolius), Asian ginseng root (Panax ginseng), licorice root.

American Ginseng Herbal Tea
Made from 100% American ginseng root, this tea has the maximum amount of this beneficial adaptogenic herb. It is used to help build the body's vitality, strength and resistance to mental and physical stress, and to help support the healthy function of the immune system. Prized by Chinese herbalists for long-term use, it was considered beneficial for fatigue and recovery from illness.

Jasmine Green Tea
Made from jasmine flowers combined with green tea, creating a delicious aromatic tea. Jasmine was traditionally used for its calming, relaxing and warming properties, for brightening the mood and as a soothing digestive tea.

100% Ginger Root Tea is a delicious and spicy tea bag that supplies a terrific boost at any time.

Also available: 100% American Ginseng Root Tea, to support balance, health and well-being.

Detox Tea
   A very gentle way to detox in a tea bag. Includes red clover, dandelion root, licorice root, peppermint leaf, ginger root, rhubarb root, burdock root and other ingredients.

   All the above is available from **Triple Leaf Tea, Inc.**

Pau d' arco
   A legendary tea from the Paraguayan rain forest which is anti-inflammatory and works well against fungal, bacterial and yeast problems. Comes in both tea bags and bulk. Available from:

Wisdom of the Ancients
1-800-899-9908
www.wisdomherbs.com

Grains

   Available from the following companies:

Lundberg Family Farms
530-882-4550 (ext. 319)
www.lundberg.com
   Grower and marketer of organic rice and rice products. They have an amazing variety of rices, rice cakes, etc. Reliable quality. Available in health food stores or order from Natural Lifestyle at 1-800-752-2775.

Omega Nutrition
1-800-661-3529
www.omeganutrition.com
Wild Rice
   Natural Canada Lake wild rice with no chemicals used. Certified organic. Available in 7oz. box or 5lb. bulk.

Organic Whole Grains
   Natural Chef Organization whole grains

High quality grains that include whole oats, spelt, barley, buckwheat and many others. It is available from:

Natural Lifestyle
1-800-752-2775
www.natural-lifestyle.com

First Lady's Lunch Bar
Contains oats, honey, almonds, sunflower seeds, dates, High Desert bee pollen, lecithin, natural flavorings (vanilla) and kelp. Available in a 1.3 oz. bar. This is a nutritious food bar with 153 calories. Available from:

Omega Nutrition
1-800-661-3529
www.omeganutrition.com

Green Drinks—Powdered and Other Specialty Powdered Drinks

For those who don't get a chance to eat the necessary amount of green vegetables we have listed four of the very best to help make up the shortage in our bodies of the necessary nutrients that are found in green products. Available from the following companies:

Jarrow Formulas™
1-800-726-0886
www.jarrow.com
Iso-Rich Soy
+ Greens
A concentrated protein powder at 462 gm strength. Two heaping tablespoons (33 g) contains Isolfavones, Glycitin, Daisin, Genistein, Chlorella, Bromelain, Papain, IP6, Spirulina, Lecithin (non-GMO). It is 100% natural. There is NO corn, yeast wheat, dairy products, preservatives or colors added. Mix 2 tablespoons of powder with 6-8 ozs fruit juice, milk or use with liquid, ice and

fruits for smoothies; mix into cold or cooked cereal or add to soups.

Garden of Life
1-800-622-8986
www.gardenoflifeuse.com
Super Green Formula
   Over forty-five nutrient dense super foods equivalent to five to ten servings of vegetables. Contains ninety antioxidants plus one hundred minerals and vitamins. Available in both powdered form and capsules.

Omega Nutrition
1-800-661-3529
www.omeganutrition.com
Bryson Greens™
   Contains a wide range of natural phytonutrients, including lignans, essential fatty acids, vitamins and minerals, a pre-biotic and probiotics, metabolic enzymes, and easily assimilated proteins. It also includes ancient sprouted grains, barley grass, broccoli sprouts, carrot juice, and Reishi and Shiitake mushrooms. Available in 10.6 oz. bottle.

NutriCology, Inc.
1-800-545-9960
www.nutricology.com
ProGreens®
   ProGreens® is a mixture of healthy and "super" green foods. It has universal appeal because it is very energizing and reduces appetite. Most people use ProGreens® as a morning wake-up drink. Energy, appetite control and detoxification can improve overall health. Contains many antioxidants. Antioxidants are general protectors invloved in immunity, inflammation control and disease prevention. Cancer and cardiovascular disease specialists say "eat more fruits and vegetables." Available in powder and capsules.

The following three powders are available from:
JarrowFormulas™
1-800-726-0886
www.jarrow.com

Berry High™
Protects vision, circulation and capillary strength. 300 gm powder available in 10.6 oz container. One scoop (8 g) contains Billberry, Blueberry Powder, Red Raspberry, Blackberry Powder, Peach Powder, Apple Fiber Powder and others. It is 100% natural and contains NO corn, yeast, wheat, dairy products, preservatives, artificial flavors, sweeteners or colors. GMO free. Suitable for vegans.

Green Defense™
Supports detoxification antioxidants in an 8.9 oz powder. Each scoop (8.5 g) contains Yaeyama Chlorella, Spirulina, Wheat Grass Juice, Barley Grass Juice, Green Kamut Juice, Quinoa, Spinach, Broccoli and many other ingredients.

Yaeyama Chlorella
1000 gm powder. Each teaspoon (5 g) contains vitamin A (from Beta Carotene), Vitamin C, Thiamin (B_1), Riboflavin, Niacin (B_3), Vitamin B_6, Vitamin B_{12}, Magnesium, Manganese, Potassium, Chlorophyll, Chlorella Growth Factor and other ingredients.

NutriCology, Inc.
1-800-545-9960
www.nutricology.com

COMPLETE IMMUNE: AN IMMUNE SUPPORT POWDER MIX THAT CAN BE USED FOR CANCER

Complete Immune is an all-in-one powdered source of vitamins and minerals along with herbs for immune support. It has been used by cancer patients before, during, and after chemotherapy and radiation. Used by cancer hospitals and clinics. Improves the immune response. Anecdotal reports indicate that patients notice more energy and improved feelings of health after short-term use. Take a full scoop with each meal. Can be used by anyone for immune enhancement.

AGED GARLIC EXTRACT

Wakunaga of America
1-800-421-2998
www.kyolic.com
Kyolic®Aged Garlic Extract (AGE)
    The most scientifically researched garlic product in the world (over 220 studies). As we mentioned earlier in this book the use of garlic in the diet is inversely related to cancer rates. Available in capsules as well as in liquid form (that can be added to food).

Mushrooms

Shiitake Mushrooms
    High grade Shiitakes in various forms. Shiitakes medicinal capabilities are being used worldwide. This mushroom may play a role in helping to alleviate illnesses such as heart disease, cancer, and AIDS. Available from:

Natural Lifestyles
1-800-752-2775
www.natural-lifestyle.com

Nuts, Nut Butters, and Seeds—Organic

    Available from the following companies:

Living Tree Community Foods
1-800-260-5534
www.livingtreecommunity.com

Organically grown nuts and nut butters, including almonds (many varieties), macadamia nuts, pine nuts, pumpkin seeds, sunflower seeds, walnut quarters, raw almond butter, raw macadamia nut butter and raw cashew butter. A new combination, which they aptly named milk of paradise is a combination of organic macadamia and cashew spread. They also stock raw honey, raw tahini, organic cranberries and a variety of dried fruits. Plus they carry dates that have not been processed with sugar and are delicious. They make their organic nut butter in small batches so they are always fresh when shipped. Available in health food stores as well as mail order.

Omega Nutrition
1-800661-3529
www.omeganutrition.com
Almonds (Raw)
Certified organically grown in California, raw almonds are an excellent source of protein, vitamins, minerals, and essential fatty acids.

Pumpkin Seed Butter
A delicious, highly nutritious spread made from grade A pumpkin seeds.

Tree Of Life
www.treeoflife.com
A company that distributes quality foods and supplements into most natural and health food stores throughout the country. They have a complete line of raw and roasted nut butters, fifteen different varieties available in natural and organic. They also have a complete line of ready-to-eat tofu and frozen organic vegetables and fruit. You can check their website for more information about their products.

Oils

Available in bottles and in gel capsules.
Recommended from the following companies:

Omega Nutrition
1-800-661-3529
www.omeganutrition.com
Essential Balance Jr. (for children)
Omega's proprietary blend of five fresh-pressed oils scientifically blended in the evolutionary 1:1 omega-3/omega-6 ratio. Contains certified organic flax, sunflower, sesame, pumpkin and borage oils. Also contains gamma-linolenic acid (GLA) and omega-6 fatty acids. Formulated with a natural butterscotch flavoring that kids will love.

Flax Seed Oil
Unrefined and certified organic, grown without pesticides or artificial fertilizers and processed using Omega's exclusive omegaflo® process. Also available from Omega Nutrition.

Olive Oil

Made from unrefined, mature organic arabequina extra-virgin olives that are fresh-pressed and omegaflo® bottled.
Also available from Omega Nutrition.

Living Tree Community Foods
1-800-260-5534
www.livingtreecommunity.com
Living Tree has a raw organic olive oil, which is not pressed. It's centrifuged at 75 degrees Fahrenheit, room temperature.

Fish Oil

Carlson Laboratories
1-800-323-4141
www.carlsonlabs.com

Norwegian Cod Liver Oil

Bottled in liquid form. This product is an effective blend of omega-3 and other essential fatty acids, as well as vitamin E. Available in natural and lemon-flavored. Can be mixed into food.

Super Omega-3 Fish Oils

Contains a special concentrate of fish body oils, from deep, coldwater fish, including mackerel and sardines, which are especially rich in EPA and DHA. Each softgel provides 570 mg of total omega-3 fatty acids consisting of EPA (Eicosapentaenoic Acid), DHA (Docosahexaenoic Acid), and ALA (Alpha-Liolenic Acid). Also available from Carlson Laboratories.

DHA Essential Fatty Acids—Omega-3

DHA, an essential fatty acid necessary for life, is available in a non-fish, micro-algae form (for those who don't want to use fish products). Look for a product called Neuromins® DHA (in softgel form). Two of the very best companies distributing Neuromins are:

Source Naturals®
1-800-815-2333

Carotec, Inc.
1-800-522-4279

Neuromins® DHA is available at health food stores.

Most poultry and fish available in this country today are loaded with unhealthy food colorings, antibiotics, hormones and many other additives the human body was not meant to absorb. For total body health it is important to use food products that are free of toxic substances. Natural products will taste even better than the products that are loaded with all kinds of artificial additives.

POULTRY

This is one of the most reliable trustworthy companies supplying additive free, free-range turkeys and chickens

Sheltons Poultry, Inc.
1-800-541-1833
www.sheltons.com
Free-range chicken and turkey with no added antibiotics. The taste quality of these natural products is far superior to products that are laced with all sorts of additives and hormones. Available in natural foods stores. Noted health expert, Andrew Weil, M.D., cautions people to avoid eating poultry and meat with added antibiotics, which has been linked to drug-resistant strains of disease-causing bacteria. Available in some health food stores.

Organic Chicken Broth
A wonderful all natural organic chicken broth with no preservatives or chemicals added. Contains organic chicken broth concentrate, sea salt, organic chicken fat, organic onion powder and organic celery seeds. Available in cans in regular and also in fat-free/sodium-free.

This company also has a wide array of other organically raised turkey and chicken, including sausage, liver and many other items. Call them for their extensive catalog.

Seafood

With all the favorable advice we are getting from our physicians about Omega 3, the following company is a reliable source for fish:

Seafood Direct
1-800-732-1836
www.seafooddirect.com
This company is a wonderful source for wild-caught salmon.

Most of the salmon available in restaurants and stores are farm-raised. Usually this means medications such as antibiotics and hormones have been added to the feed, as well as synthetic coloring. Wild-caught salmon has none of these problems and a high level of omega-3 fatty acids and much less fat than farm-raised salmon. It tastes better as well. Their line includes Wild Alaskan Salmon, King Salmon and Sockeye Salmon. Alaskan caught King Crab, Crab and Alaskan Cod are also available. They come in frozen filets and steaks. Also in jars and cans. An excellent canned salmon and canned solid white albacore tuna, which is caught with hook and line to guarantee quality, are also available. Again there are no added preservatives. Available in some health food and gourmet stores.

Stevia

Omega Nutrition
1-800-661-3529
www.omeganutrition.com

Stevia Powdered Crystals
This powder is pure stevia extract using certified organic leaves and a patented water filtration process. 1 oz. container.

Stevia Supreme Packets
A mix of stevia and erythritol (natural filler) put into convenient packets. Unlike other fillers, erythritol is easily digested, dissolves quickly, is safe for diabetics, and has no calories or carbohydrates. Each box of Stevia Supreme Packets contains 50 packets.

Wisdom of the Ancients®
1-800-899-9908
www.wisdomherbs.com
Natural sweetener made from whole leaf Stevia (*Stevia rebaudiana Bertoni*) 6:1 concentrated extract. Available in concentrated tablets, liquid, and as a tea. Hundreds of scientific studies

have been conducted on Stevia's effectiveness as a nutritional addition to the diet.

Wine—Organic

The following wine company is outstanding, not only because of the quality and good taste of their wines, but they are also one of the very few who do not add sulfites, which can have an adverse affect on many people.

Frey Vineyards
1-800-760-3739
or call their distributor: (they will help you find a local store that carries this brand).

Organic Vintages
877-ORGANIC
If you enjoy an occasional glass of wine, we strongly suggest avoidance of pesticides and other chemicals. Frey Vineyards is a fine and reliable certified organic wine company. They do not add sulfites to their wine.

Dental Products

There is a holistic connection between the health of your teeth and gums and your whole body. This is especially true for diabetics, who need to be vigilant about their teeth and gums because they have a tendency to develop periodontal disease. Woodstock Natural Products are formulated by a holistic dentist and contain soothing and healing herbs, with no alcohol, sugar, or harsh chemicals. These products have been clinically proven to kill germs that cause gum disease. In a study published in the *Journal of Clinical Dentistry* in 1998, researchers at the New York University College of Dentistry in New York City found that The Natural Dentist toothpaste removed plaque more effectively than the leading commercial brand. The same group also found that The Natural Dentist mouth rinse killed more germs than the leading commercial brand.

Woodstock Natural Products, Inc.
The Natural Dentist™
1-800-615-6895
Toothpaste: mint, cinnamon and fluoride-free mint
Mouth rinse: mint, cinnamon, and cherry-flavored
Available in health food stores.

Desert Essence®
1-800-476-8647
www.desertessence.com
Oral Care Collection
   A complete line of antiseptic and cleansing oral care products using tea tree oil for deep cleaning and disinfecting of teeth and gums. All products are animal and eco-friendly and made without artificial colors, sweeteners or harsh abrasives.

Tea Tree Oil Dental Floss: creates a germ-free mouth and cleans between teeth.
Tea Tree Oil Dental Tape: provides same benefits as floss with a wider ribbon.
Tea Tree Oil Dental Pics: cleans between teeth with antiseptic power.
Tea Tree Oil Breath Freshener: contains natural and organic essential oils.

ENVIRONMENT

Environmentally Safe Toxin Free Cleansers
   Toxic chemicals can play a very significant role in causing a variety of illnesses.

   There are many dangerous and toxic chemicals that can migrate into the human body. An easy way to keep some of them away is to avoid commercial brands of cleansers. There are several excellent companies that market effective cleansers and do not contain harmful chemicals. Here are two of the very best.

Earth Friendly Products
1-800-335-3267 Ext. 10
www.ecos.com

Stain & Odor Remover
    An effective non-polluting 100% biodegradable cleanser for removing all sorts of stains and dirt. This product will work on carpets, fabrics, clothing, laundry, wood floors and other surfaces.

The Wave Automatic Machine Dishwashing Powder. (Also available in gel form)
    A very effective non-toxic cleanser. Chlorine-free and phosphate-free.

ECOS®
A toxic-free liquid or powder washing machine cleanser.

    Earth Friendly Products also has a variety of other products including window cleaner, all purpose cleansers and even a drain opener and maintainer made with enzymes. Available in health food stores.

Allens Naturally
1-800-352-8971
www.allensnaturally.com
    All of the cleansing products at this company are free of perfume and dyes, are biodegradable and very powerful. They have a long list of natural cleansers ranging from dishwasher and washing machine cleanser, as well as glass and several all-purpose cleansers. Available in health food stores or can be obtained from N.E.E.D.S at 1-800-634-1380.

Environmental Products

Mail Order

N.E.E.D.S
1-800-634-1380
www.needs.com
   An excellent resource for top-notch environmental products.
Call them for a full listing of their products.

Aireox Home Purifer (Model 45)
   Removes mold spores, pollen dust, formaldehyde, and more.

Aireox Car Air Purifier (Model 22)
   An unusual purifier for the car.

Allens Naturally
   A full line of toxin-free household cleansers, including dishwashing and laundry detergents and all-purpose cleaners.

Water Filters
   N.E.E.D.S. carries a variety of high-quality water filters.

Elite Shower Filter and Massager
   For removing chlorine, heavy metals and bacteria. The amount
of chlorine that can penetrate the skin while taking a shower is
substantial. Chlorine is a toxin, which can cause damage to body
tissues.

Environmental Pressure Cooker
SILIT Pressure Cooker

   Most cooking appliances use an aluminum cooking surface.
This metal is very inexpensive for the manufacturer, but the user
must beware, aluminum can cause toxic reactions in the human
body. More expensive appliances will use stainless steel. However, there are several other metals within stainless steel. One of

which is nickel, which again, when absorbed by the body can set off toxic reactions.

An ideal cooking surface is enamel. This is much like glassware, but is not breakable and has no known toxic materials. A wonderful new pressure cooker using an enamel surface is now available. This sophisticated device has new controls, which automatically controls steam to avoid burns, while at the same time retaining all the natural flavors and nutrients within food. This superb cooker enhances the taste with aromatic steam because of its patented hermetically sealed system. It will cook most everything safely and much quicker than most cooking systems. Available from:

Natural Lifestyle
1-800-752-2775
www.natural-lifestyle.com

WATER

Water is the forgotten element in our daily lives. We forget or do not realize, that the human body can survive for weeks without food. But this is not the reality of water. Without water, our survival time is limited to at best a few days. We usually have at our disposal municipal supplied water, which may be subject to contamination. Or we can carefully choose bottled water, which is now a multibillion dollar industry. There are dozens of brands available. Some of which are no more than processed water, obtained from regular municipal water supplies.

Making a choice: Consider the source. The best water will be obtained from protected spring waters that are contaminant-free and bottled under stringent quality control procedures at the natural source. Ideally, this water would be available in pure glass bottles or containers, which unlike some plastic bottles will not leak dangerous chemicals into the body. Additionally, water should be sodium-free, contain important minerals and hopefully be slightly alkaline rather than acidic.

One of the very best having all of these qualifications is the following:

Mountain Valley Spring Water
1-800-643-1501
www.mountainvalleyspring.com
This water company has been bottling and distributing their pure, delicious spring water since 1871. They are one of the few bottled waters that still offer their product in glass.

Purified Water

It is often thought that distilled drinking water is the purest of all water. But, distilled has no minerals for the body's use. Now a new and improved water is even purer than distilled or even reverse osmosis water. This product has less than 0.4 PPM or 25 times less dissolved solids than either distilled or reverse osmosis.

Penta™ Purified Drinking Water
1-800-531-5088
www.hydrateforlife.com

We have been advised by some of the doctors about some new and very effective **supplements.**

OLIVE LEAF EXTRACT

Seagate (also known as First Fishery)
1-888-505-4283
www.seagateproducts.com
As we enter a new millennium, antibiotics are no longer seen as a risk-free panacea. Their rampant overuse has created resistant strains of bacteria that are not so easy to treat. Antibiotics

have also been found to have serious side effects such as allergic reactions, colitis and yeast overgrowth. The olive leaf and its extract have been used for thousands of years against almost all pathological microorganisms, including fungi, bacteria, viruses, parasites and other microscopic organisms. There has been increasing interest in the use of natural anti-microbial products in recent years as a result of the increasing awareness of the public to the side effects of pharmaceutical drugs and their reduced ability to combat the evolving mutant strains of these microorganisms.

Olive Leaf Extract has been used safely for thousands of years by people along the Mediterranean Sea. This is a natural plant product, not a drug. The only known side effect that has been noted from the use of Olive Leaf Extract is the possibility of a Herxheimer reaction—which is the rapid die-off of a large number of harmful fungi that suddenly release toxins, which then may trigger an immune response, similar to an allergic or flu-like reaction, for a few days. If this reaction is experienced and becomes too uncomfortable, the level of use can be reduced or stopped until the reaction disappears. Some doctors believe that a Herxheimer reaction is an excellent response for an anti-fungal treatment.

For therapeutic use, take 4–9 capsules per day. As a natural antimicrobial health food supplement, for most applications (other than fungal disorders) the suggested use is three capsules three times per day for a week to ten days. For antifungal support, the suggested use is two capsules three times per day for up to six months; or in more severe cases, up to twelve months. Olive Leaf Extract is available in fine health food stores.

Shark Liver Oil (also available from Seagate)
    This particular Shark Liver Oil has a 30% composition of Omega-3 fatty acids, which includes EPA (eicosapentaenoic acid—9.1%) and DHA (docosahexaenoic acid—16.1%). This oil also contains trace amounts of squalene. Available in soft gel capsules.

Resurgex™

Among anti-oxidants, the Superoxide Dismutase (SOD) enzyme family appears to be among the most potent system to revitalize and reduce the rate of cell destruction. It promotes the removal of the super-oxide (one of the most potent free radicals in the body). Recently a French company has discovered a unique delivery system for SOD that has proven to be most effective in delivering this critically important enzyme in the body. This product comes in a powdered form and the major ingredient is SOD/Gliadin. It is available from:

Millennium Biotechnologies, Inc.
1-908-630-8700
www.milbiotech.com

BioCalth®/Calcium L-Threonate™

Many doctors recommend the use of BioCalth® as a primary source of calcium and collagen regeneration. Unfortunately calcium supplements for the most part, that are sold in the U.S. market today, are not properly absorbed by the body. The National Osteoporosis Foundation describes bones as composed of "a protein framework." This protein framework is a collagen matrix that allows minerals such as calcium to attach. Without the foundation and flexibility of collagen, the bones will be brittle as in Osteoporosis and the cartilage at the joints will still be worn out as in Osteoporosis. Scientific studies have shown that BioCalth® promotes bone collagen synthesis by elevating the body's ability to produce collagen. The patented BioCalth® promotes healthy production of collagen in the body. The calcium in BioCalth® is 95% absorbed, which means it is an important addition to the diet of individuals who want to improve the balance between bone formation and reabsorption. No other calcium will lay down a bed of collagen; this is important because without a new bed of collagen the calcium is unable to build new bone. BioCalth® is significantly effective for the reduction of pain, cramps, and weakness in the limbs and the body, as well as reducing the risks of bone fractures, Osteoporosis and Osteoarthritis. For further information on this product, please contact:

BioCalth International Corp.
1871 Wright Avenue
LaVerne, CA 91750
1-888-275-1717
www.biocalth.com

Cleartrac™
This is a natural probiotic fiber which acts as a food source for the growth of beneficial bacteria in the gastrointestinal tract. It is derived from a natural substance from the larex tree and contains specially formulated arabinogalactan, a natural occurring botanical extract. It comes in a powdered form and is available from:

Larex Inc.
1-800-386-5300
www.larex.com

The following are available from:

NutriCology, Inc.
1-800-545-9960
www.nutricology.com

AngioBlock
AngioBlock is a natural extract of bindweek or *Convolvulus arvensis*. Studies have shown AngioBlock to induce angiogenesis inhibition (angiogenesis is a tumor's ability to develop a blood supply for growth). It is a water extraction of the leaves of the herb and is rich in proteoglycan mixture (PGM). In combination with proper nutrition, it can enhance the immune system's ability to maintain good health and resist disease. Available in capsules.

IndoleGard

A new and important supplement that has been shown to support the body in healthy estrogen metabolism and hormone regulation. Contains BioResponseDIM™, a formulation of pure dietary indole from cruciferous vegetables available from Nutri-Cology. Available in capsules.

Ovary Prostate Health

Ovary Prostate health is a mixture of four Chinese and Vietnamese herbs supportive to the immune system, the prostate and ovaries. The combination of these herbs in the present formulation originates from medical insights resulting from a unique application of Oriental medicine, and traces back over a number of generations. Interestingly enough, it seems to support the health of both the prostate and the ovaries. Available in tablets.

Index